EAT FOR LONGEVITY—
YOU'RE ONLY AS OLD AS YOU FEEL!

- **Being carb and sugar smart**

- **Balancing good and bad fats to slow down your body clock**

- **Making fiber your friend**

- **Calcium and antioxidants— everything you need to know**

- **Exercising your brain and your body**

- **What to eat—and delicious ways to eat it!**

- **An essential, age-defying nutrition counter . . . AND MORE!**

FOODS THAT COMBAT AGING

Foods That
COMBAT
AGING

The Nutritional
Way to Stay Healthy
Longer

DEBORAH MITCHELL

A Lynn Sonberg Book

HARPER

An Imprint of HarperCollinsPublishers

HARPER

An Imprint of HarperCollins*Publishers*
10 East 53rd Street
New York, New York 10022-5299

First Harper paperback printing: January 2008

HarperCollins® and Harper® are registered trademarks of Harper-Collins Publishers.

Printed in the United States of America

Visit Harper paperbacks on the World Wide Web at
www.harpercollins.com

10 9 8 7 6 5 4 3 2 1

CONTENTS

INTRODUCTION

Getting older sure beats the alternative, so the saying goes, but must we have such a gloomy, defeatist attitude about aging? Absolutely not! In fact, there are many things you can do *right now, every day*, to help minimize the effects of aging while you grow older.

There's no denying it: growing older is a natural part of the life cycle. From the moment you were conceived, you began to age. The years keep passing, and there's no turning back. The secret is in how you make the journey, and a big part of the trip involves food. You can make nutrition and lifestyle choices that promote health, longevity, and vitality, or those that make you feel, look, and act old. The choice is up to you.

Some older men and women proudly proclaim that they are having the best times of their lives, that they can finally do things when, how, where, if, and with whom they want. For them, and indeed for the majority of people, the older years can mean a chance to travel, explore new hobbies, go back to school, volunteer for a favorite cause, even start a new career.

Yet our negative and fearful attitudes about getting older are grounded in some real concerns, and one of the main ones is this: Will we be physically, mentally, and emotionally capable of enjoying the decades of life ahead of us? This is a legitimate question, and one that you as an adult, *regardless of your age*, should think about and address now to help make the most of your older years.

Foods That Combat Aging can help you make positive food and nutrition choices that combat aging every day and help you maintain health, vitality, and a positive attitude that helps you enjoy life. The great thing about making food choices that help fight aging is that you get several chances every day to make a positive impact on your health and your fight against aging. And if you make a not-so-great selection or two once in a while, you know that you can go right back to making great choices at your next meal!

SIGNS AND SYMPTOMS OF AGING

Hair turns gray, energy flags, fine wrinkles appear, and house keys get misplaced a little more often—these are just a few indications of growing older. Everyone ages differently; the number of signs and symptoms, their severity, when they appear, how they respond to our attempts to reduce or eliminate them—all of these factors and more should be considered when you talk about aging and how to combat it. The list of changes associated with aging is a long one, but here is a representative look.

- General decrease in energy level and a tendency to tire easily
- Decreased memory
- Decreased sex drive
- Abdominal obesity and an inability to lose weight
- Some hearing loss, especially for higher frequencies
- Development of arthritis: affects about one-third of men and one-half of women
- Loss of lean muscle tissue
- Development of insulin resistance
- Changes in bowel function
- Changes in hair color and volume
- Tendency to sleep more lightly and to experience less rapid eye movement (REM) sleep
- Reduction in muscle strength
- Reduction in bone density
- Reduction in reaction time
- Reduction in levels of antibodies (and thus ability to fight off infections)
- Reduction in levels of most hormones

There is much you can do to reduce, compensate for, or slow the progression of many of these and other physical and metabolic changes that occur with aging. One of the most important things you can do is harness the power of anti-aging nutrition, which we do in two ways in this book. One is through the convenient anti-aging nutrition counter offered in the second part of this book. The other is through a discussion of the dietary steps and other actions that complement any nutritional efforts you take in your fight against aging. Let's look at some of these other approaches, along with a discussion of how wise food and supplement choices can help you *fight aging now!*

CHAPTER 1

FIGHT AGING NOW

You are fortunate to live in a time when the field of anti-aging medicine has become a vital and increasingly well-researched area of medicine. Health-care practitioners who are involved in anti-aging medicine are excited by the forward-thinking nature of this new approach, which involves helping people take the steps necessary to maximize quality of life in their later years. Basically, anti-aging medicine is concerned with three concepts.

- Prevention: taking steps to prevent the development of diseases and ailments associated with growing older. Proper nutrition is a key element of prevention.
- Integration: combining the best of both worlds—conventional and alternative/complementary medicine—to achieve anti-aging goals.

- Holism: recognizing and treating people as whole beings composed of many integrated parts that work together. Thus an anti-aging approach to arthritis of the hip addresses all the factors that have an impact on arthritis, including diet, exercise level, social needs, stress management, emotional health, supplementation, and pharmaceuticals.

EAT FOR LONGEVITY

Three or more times a day, you have a chance to fight aging with food! Your food choices are one of the most important ways you impact your health, and so it's vitally important that you understand the basics behind what makes certain foods good partners in the fight against aging. We say "partners" because although healthy food choices are key purely on a nutritional level, they also work hand-in-hand with other factors in the effort to ward off aging, namely, exercise, stress management, supplementation, and hormone balancing. In this book we focus on nutrition, but in this chapter we also explain the relationship between wise food choices and these other factors that impact aging.

BE SUGAR SMART

This section could be called "Be Carb Smart," but we want to impress upon you that when we talk about carbohydrates, we're really talking about sugars.

That's because *all carbohydrates are broken down (metabolized) into simple sugars.* Therefore, because sugars are the bottom line when it comes to carbohydrates and their metabolism, we think it's important to begin there. Once you see the connection between carbs and aging, you'll never look at carbs quite the same way again. Here's the story.

Carbs come in two forms: simple or refined, and complex. Simple sugars include table sugar and natural sugars found in fruits, honey, and milk. Refined carbs are in white flour, white rice, baked goods, and refined pasta. Simple/refined sugars not only get stored as fat if you eat too much of them, but they also cause blood glucose levels to rise. Elevated blood glucose levels, especially chronically, can lead to insulin resistance (when the body cannot produce enough insulin or cannot adequately use the insulin it does produce) and eventually result in diabetes and its many complications, including heart disease, kidney disease, nerve disorders, and blindness.

But the link between carbs and aging is this: high blood glucose (sugar) levels accelerate aging through a process called glycation. Glycation is a natural occurrence in which glucose molecules and certain fat molecules interact with and attach to protein molecules, forming AGEs—advanced glycation end-products—and damage the protein. Wrinkling of skin is one example of what glycation can do, as collagen and other proteins in skin are damaged by glucose. Although glycation occurs in everyone, it speeds up when there's a lot of glucose present. The rest of the bad news is that glycation is not reversible, so the goal is to prevent it as much as possible. How do you do that?

What You Can Do Now

You can be sugar smart and keep your blood glucose levels in a healthy range (ideally, a fasting glucose level that is less than 100 mg/dL). Since carbohydrates are a key energy source, you need to provide your body with the best fuel in the form of smart carbs—complex carbs rather than simple ones. Complex carbs are more complicated in structure and generally higher in nutritional value than simple carbs. A diet that includes a moderate amount of carbs (about 50% of total caloric intake), mostly the complex type, can help keep blood glucose levels in check, as complex carbs generally cause a moderate increase in blood glucose levels while simple ones cause a sharp, rapid (and unhealthy) rise.

Another factor to consider is the glycemic index, which is a gauge of how quickly foods convert into glucose. Foods with a low value (generally 50 or lower) convert into glucose slower, which keeps blood glucose levels more balanced throughout the day and thus helps fight aging. Here are some smart carb tips, followed by a sample glycemic index.

- Choose brown or wild rice instead of white rice.
- Substitute whole-wheat or other whole-grain breads, rolls, and bagels for their white flour cousins.

- Include one to two servings (½ cup per serving) of beans daily: lima, butter, white, pinto, black, soy, kidney, or garbanzo.
- Choose yams or sweet potatoes instead of white potatoes.
- Include one serving of oatmeal or all-bran cereal daily.
- Choose whole fresh fruits for dessert.
- Choose a whole-grain pasta (wheat, spelt, buckwheat, rye) instead of white pasta.
- Significantly reduce or eliminate white sugar and white sugar products from your diet.
- If you use fruit juices or fruit products, choose unsweetened varieties: unsweetened apple sauce, juices and nectars, canned or jarred fruits (in natural juices only).

GOOD FAT/BAD FAT

It's become common practice to classify fat into two categories—"good" and "bad"—to make it easier to identify which ones you should include more of in your diet and which ones to reduce or avoid. Certainly when we talk about fighting aging, we want to optimize the benefits of good fats and minimize the damage from the bad ones.

First you should understand that "fat" comes in four main types: saturated, polyunsaturated (which includes omega-3 and omega-6), monounsaturated, and trans fats. Fat is essential for life: most of the body's organs—especially the brain—could not function without it. But "essential" does not mean you need large amounts of it. Although the Dietary Guidelines recommend Americans consume 20 to 35 percent of their calories from fat, the lower end of that range is much healthier and realistic given that the majority of people in the United States are overweight or obese and that diseases associated with high-fat intake (e.g., heart disease, stroke, some cancers) are responsible for the majority of disease-related deaths.

"Good fats" include monounsaturated fats and omega-3 fatty acids, a type of polyunsaturated fat. These fats typically are not listed on nutrition labels and so information about their values in foods is usually not readily available. You can calculate the amount of good fat in a product by subtracting the sum of bad fats from the total fat value. The resulting number is a fairly accurate idea of the amount of good fat in the product, although the figure may also represent some of the polyunsaturated fat called omega-6, which is sometimes good, sometimes bad. In the nutrition counter in this book, we provide values for total fat, bad fats, and good fats.

Although fats can have many negative effects on your health and contribute to aging, they also have many anti-aging benefits if you eat the right ones. That's why it's important to eat a balanced amount of good and bad fats. What does that mean? Your intake of bad fats should be less than 10 percent of your total caloric intake, and your intake of good fats should be at least 15 percent to 20 percent of your total caloric intake. Based on a 2,000 calorie per day diet, less than 200 calories should come from bad fats, and 300 to 400 should come from good fats. You should remember that all fats provide 9 calories per gram, which is more than twice as much as the calories supplied by carbohydrates and protein (4 per gram). So if you order a fast-food fish sandwich that has 15 grams of saturated fat and 2 grams of trans fat, you've nearly reached your daily limit for bad fats with one food item alone ($9 \times 17 = 153$ g).

So what are some of the benefits of eating a balanced amount of good and bad fats?

- They help the body absorb the fat-soluble vitamins (A, D, E, and K). This ability declines with aging.
- They make you feel fuller, which helps you resist the temptation to eat between meals and before bed.
- They help keep the brain healthy. The brain is composed of 60 percent fat, and if you deprive your body of a sufficient amount of good dietary fats, symptoms associated with aging, such as poor concentration, faulty memory, and reduced acuity, are likely to occur and with greater severity.
- They help keep the immune system operating optimally so it can fight off infection, promote wound healing, and reduce the risk of cancer.

- Age-related changes to skin, hair, and nails can be reduced.
- Fats help the gastrointestinal system avoid constipation, bloating, and other digestive problems that are common as we age.
- A small amount of saturated fat is needed by the liver to manufacture cholesterol, which the body uses to produce hormones. Restoration of declining hormone levels, which occurs with age, is an important factor in the fight against aging (see "Balancing Hormones").
- Fats help maintain a healthy nervous system.

Good sources of monounsaturated fats and omega-3 fatty acids include olive oil, avocadoes, salmon, walnuts, herring, and olives.

Bad Fats

Bad fats include saturated fat, which is most often found in animal products, including meats, poultry, fish, and dairy products, as well as some tropical oils, such as palm and coconut; and trans fat, an artificial fat created when an unsaturated fat is bombarded with hydrogen atoms, resulting in a partially saturated fat.

Bad fats contribute to aging in a big way, namely:

- Saturated fats increase the amount of "bad" cholesterol (low-density lipoprotein, LDL) in the bloodstream, which causes heart disease, atherosclerosis, and restricted blood flow.

- Saturated fats are associated with insulin resistance, a leading cause of diabetes.
- Both saturated fat and trans fat are associated with an increased risk of colon cancer.
- Eating trans fat doubles the risk of heart attack by increasing the levels of LDL cholesterol, decreasing the levels of HDL (high-density lipoprotein) cholesterol (the "good" cholesterol), and promoting the formation of blood clots, all of which increase the risk of heart attack and stroke.
- Trans fat increases triglyceride levels, which increases the risk of developing blood clots.
- Trans fat causes inflammation of blood vessels by increasing levels of C-reactive protein, which in turn increases the risk of heart disease.
- Liver function, the immune system, and reproductive function are all harmed by the consumption of trans fat.

What You Can Do Now

A diet high in saturated and trans fat is associated with elevated blood cholesterol levels, which can result in heart disease and other serious medical conditions. The nutrition counter in this book can help you identify the amount of bad fats in foods so you can make healthier choices. You can also reduce the amount of bad fats in your diet if you:

- eat more fruits, vegetables, and whole grains.
- choose non-fat and low-fat dairy products.

- remove the skin from poultry.
- steam and sauté foods rather than fry them.
- limit meat consumption to lean cuts while avoiding organ meats.
- regularly substitute plant protein for animal protein (e.g., beans, peas, lentils, tofu, tempeh).
- read ingredient labels and avoid foods that contain trans fats, which appear as "partially hydrogenated vegetable oil," "hydrogenated oil," or "margarine." Baked goods, crackers and cookies, processed and frozen dinners, fried foods, and margarines typically contain trans fats.

MAKE FIBER YOUR FRIEND

Remember when the word "fiber" used to make people snicker and look embarrassed? People aren't snickering anymore, because they're learning just how important fiber is and how getting enough of it can not only make you feel better, but live healthier, longer.

Fiber is a calorie-free nutrient that is necessary for maintaining regular bowel movements, controlling cholesterol and blood glucose levels, and helping with weight loss or maintenance. It has been shown to help reduce the risk of colon cancer, one of the primary causes of cancer death in the United States.

Fiber is present in food in two forms: soluble fiber, which is a sticky type found mostly in beans, dried peas, oats, nuts, seeds, and most fruits, such as apricots, bananas, grapes, and citrus. Soluble fiber is responsible for normalizing blood glucose levels and reducing cholesterol levels in the blood. Insoluble fiber is coarse and helps promote intestinal regularity. It is found mainly in vegetables, bran cereals, wheat bran, whole-grain cereals, and pears.

What You Can Do Now

Most adults consume about half of the recommended amount of fiber, which is 38 grams for males 19 to 50 years of age and 25 grams for women of the same age. It is important to get the recommended amount of fiber daily to help prevent age-related diseases, such as heart disease, diabetes, and atherosclerosis, and to help maintain skin health. Here are a few tips on how to increase your fiber intake. The nutrition counter in the back of the book also contains information on fiber content of more than 3,000 foods.

- Choose whole-grain breads, rolls, and pastas instead of those made with white flour.
- When appropriate, eat the skins of fruits and vegetables. Buy organic produce when possible, and always thoroughly wash produce before eating it.
- "Sneak" extra fiber into your diet: sprinkle a tablespoon of wheat germ on your cereal, choose

granola for a snack instead of chips, add flax seeds and kidney beans to your salad.

- Choose bean dip instead of those made with sour cream. Serve the dip with raw vegetables instead of chips.
- Include one serving of beans, lentils, or split peas per day. These can be in chili, soups, stews, salads, or as a side dish.
- Include one serving of oatmeal, all-bran, or another high-fiber cereal per day.

CALCIUM

There's no bones about it, you need adequate amounts of calcium to keep your bones healthy. Calcium is especially critical for bone health, and for the 44 million Americans for whom osteoporosis is a major health threat. The National Institutes of Arthritis and Musculoskeletal and Skin Diseases reports that 10 million Americans already have osteoporosis and 34 million more are at increased risk for the disease. Of special concern is the fact that 50% of women and 25% of men older than 50 will experience an osteoporosis-related fracture during their lifetime, contributing to the more than 1.5 million osteoporosis-related fractures that occur each year. Osteoporosis can also cause pain and limit mobility and thus have a negative impact on the quality of life.

Calcium is essential for more than bone health. This mineral also protects against colon cancer, is key to dental health, aids in the production of energy, and is critical for heart and nerve function.

National surveys show that many Americans consume less than 50% of the calcium they need. Because calcium needs change over a lifetime, many people forget to ensure they are getting enough of this critical mineral. As people age, the body becomes less efficient at absorbing calcium, and this problem is compounded by the fact that many older adults take medications that can impair calcium absorption. The need for more calcium also kicks in for both older men and women who are postmenopausal.

What You Can Do Now

According to the Institutes of Medicine, the recommended daily intake of calcium for both men and women is 1,000 mg daily for adults 31 to 50 years, and 1,200 mg for those older than 50. Vitamin D is essential for calcium absorption, so try to get 400 to 600 IU (international units) per day up to age 70, and up to 800 IU if you are 70 or older. Here are some ways to ensure you get enough calcium.

- Dairy foods can be a good source of calcium, but they also contain a lot of protein (see warning in bullet below). If you eat dairy products, include low-fat varieties.
- Many non-dairy foods are also very good sources of calcium, including dark green, leafy

vegetables such as bok choy, spinach, broccoli, and kale; sardines (with the bones) and salmon; tofu; and almonds.

- Calcium in orange juice? You bet! Many foods are now fortified with calcium, including many brands of orange juice, cereals, breads, soy milk and soy cheese.

- Moderate your protein intake. A diet that contains excess protein (many Americans consume too much protein, especially from animal sources) can contribute to the development of osteoporosis, because when excess protein leaves the body it often carries calcium with it. The World Health Organization recommends 0.45 grams of protein per kilogram (2.2 lbs) of ideal body weight per day, while the U.S. RDA recommends 0.8 grams as the maximum. Thus, if your ideal weight is 130 pounds, your minimum protein intake should be 27 grams and the maximum, 48 grams.

ADD ANTIOXIDANTS

Some of the most powerful weapons you have against aging are antioxidants—certain vitamins, minerals, and enzymes that take on free radicals and combat the extensive harm they can cause to the body. Some common and powerful antioxidants include vitamin A, C, E, B6, and B12, beta-carotene, and folic acid. Other potent antioxidants include phytonutrients, which are special chemicals found in plants.

As your body metabolizes food through a process known as oxidation, it also produces nasty by-products called free radicals. Free radicals are unstable molecules that can cause significant damage to the body's tissues and contribute to aging (including wrinkled skin) and certain diseases, such as diabetes, Alzheimer's disease, stroke, macular degeneration, and heart disease. Thus one goal of an anti-aging food plan is to include lots of antioxidants.

One important thing to remember about antioxidants is that they work best as a team: consuming many antioxidants is much more effective than using just one. One of the best ways to get a wide variety of antioxidants is to eat many different fruits and vegetables, which are naturally rich in antioxidants.

What You Can Do Now

- Eat about nine servings of fruits and vegetables daily. The 2005 US Dietary Guidelines recommend 5 to 13 servings daily, with the numbers adjusting according to the total number of calories consumed. Nine servings are recommended for a 2,000 calorie per day diet.
- When you want something sweet, reach for a piece of fruit. Or try some variety: slice up a fresh apple and pear, add some orange or tangerine

slices, a handful of berries, and squeeze some lemon juice on the mixture. This is a great snack, dessert, or a complement to your breakfast.

- Introduce more vegetables into your menu by adding chopped favorites to stews, soups, or stir-fry.
- Include a salad on your menu every day, and be creative. Try several different types of lettuce and spinach as your base, and then add shredded carrots, radishes, daikon, and red cabbage, toss in cooked string beans and peas, brighten it with chopped beets and avocado slices, and top it off with chopped walnuts and slices of red onion.
- Stuff vegetables with vegetables! Acorn and butternut squash, green and red peppers, large tomatoes, and cabbage leaves can be stuffed with a mixture of steamed and seasoned vegetables mixed with brown rice, barley, or beans.

COOK TO FIGHT AGING

It's not always *what* you eat as much as *how* you prepare it that can make a difference when it comes to aging. Remember when we talked about glycation and AGEs under "Be Sugar Smart"? AGEs are formed in the presence of high temperatures and without water, as in foods that are fried, baked, grilled, broiled, or microwaved. Thus fried foods (e.g., French fries, deep-fried fish, and vegetables), grilled chicken, baked bread, broiled steaks, fried eggs, and microwaved potatoes all contain AGEs. Although it isn't possible to completely avoid AGEs (remember, the body produces them naturally as well), you can do some things to significantly reduce your exposure to them.

What You Can Do Now

- When having fish, try poaching or steaming.
- Meats can be stewed, stir-fried, or made in a slow cooker.
- Limit the number of high-temperature foods you eat per week. If you currently eat such foods at least once a day, gradually reduce that number to once or twice a week at most.
- Steam, boil, or stir-fry vegetables, or use a slow cooker.
- Add more fresh and raw fruits and vegetables to your diet.
- Marinate foods in olive oil, mustard, garlic, lemon juice, dry wine, or cider vinegar, which reduces the formation of AGEs.

CALORIE RESTRICTION

An increasing number of studies indicate that calorie restriction extends life in both animals and humans. Studies, beginning with the first one done at Cornell University in 1935, show that the lives of many different animals can be extended 30 to 40 percent and that age-related illnesses can be delayed when their caloric intake is restricted. Today, organizations such as the American Diabetes Foundation, the National Institutes for Health and Aging, and the American Heart Association are all doing research into calorie restriction and its impact on health.

According to a study published in the *Journal of the American Medical Association*, people who followed a calorie-restricted diet for six months experienced a 24 to 25 percent decrease in body fat, a decrease in DNA damage (which occurs with aging and contributes to disease processes such as cancer), and reduced both core body temperature and fasting insulin levels, two indicators of longevity. Overall, the changes experienced by the people on a calorie-restricted diet suggest that long-term calorie restriction may extend lifespan.

What You Can Do Now

Does calorie restriction mean you have to starve if you want to live longer? Not at all. The idea behind calorie restriction is to follow a low-calorie diet but to eat nutrient-rich foods; that is, you make every calorie count! Here are some tips on how to do it.

- Include lots of high-fiber vegetables in your diet, and eat them raw when feasible.
- Focus on monounsaturated fats and omega-3 fatty acids rather than saturated and/or trans fats.
- Choose lean animal protein (including egg whites) and especially plant-based protein, which

is typically much lower in fat than animal protein. Beans, legumes, tofu, and tempeh are protein-rich plant sources.

- Choose whole, fresh fruits rather than fruit juices, which are higher in calories and sugar and have less fiber than whole fruits.
- Choose whole-grain breads, cereals, and pasta rather than those made with refined flours.
- Avoid sugar and sugary foods, processed foods, and fried foods.

Experts and those who follow a calorie restrictive approach emphasize that it is a lifestyle, not a fad diet or a short-term approach. You can learn more about calorie restriction for longevity in the "References" section at the end of this book.

EXERCISE

Wait, don't turn the page just because you see the "E" word. Study after study shows similar results: if you want to slow the aging process, you need to exercise. In a study of nearly ten thousand men ages 20 to 82 who were followed for about five years, for example, researchers found that physically unfit men who subsequently got in shape had a 44 percent lower death rate than those men who remained inactive.

Do you think you're too old to exercise? Nonsense! In a study published in the *Journal of Aging and Health* (2006), researchers reported on the exercise activities of 64 men and women ages 66 to 96 who lived in an independent living facility. The volunteers were divided into three groups: a walking group, a resistance training group, and a control group (no exercise). At the end of the sixteen-week study, the investigators found that the volunteers in both of the exercise groups enjoyed better body strength, flexibility, and agility, even in areas that were not trained, than the non-exercise group. These improvements typically translate into people being able to take better care of themselves and to live longer, healthier, more fulfilling lives. The study findings suggest that exercise in older people may provide more overall health benefits and less exercise-specific advantages than in younger people, which translates into a great deal for older adults.

What You Can Do Now

Before you start any exercise program, you should check with your doctor to make sure you choose the safest and most efficient type and intensity of exercise program for you. Moderate, regular (30 to 45 minutes, five to six days per week) exercise is the general prescription to combat aging. Remember the list of signs and symptoms of aging mentioned earlier in the book? Exercise helps fight many of them. For example, regular exercise helps improve heart and lung function, increases bone density, reduces body fat, improves muscle strength, improves the ability of the body to utilize insulin, reduces blood pressure, alleviates stress, improves mood, enhances sex drive and sexual function, and reduces joint pain.

One of the most common complaints about exercise is that it's boring, and boredom quickly leads to non-compliance. But exercise can be much more interesting if you add variety, and variety begins with a three-part approach to anti-aging exercise: stretching, aerobic training, and strength/resistance training. There are dozens of excellent books that contain suggestions and instructions in each of these categories. Always check with your doctor first, however.

- **Stretching.** It's important to maintain flexibility, and stretching is a great way to do it. Every exercise session should include stretching, but don't start your sessions with a stretch! Warm up your muscles first with five or ten minutes of moderate activity such as brisk walking. Stretching cold muscles can result in injury. After you do your aerobic and/or resistance training, then take five minutes to stretch again. Many yoga poses are excellent ways to stretch and stay flexible.
- **Aerobic training.** Choose from activities that fit your interest and abilities, such as brisk walking, jogging, swimming, biking, tennis, racquetball, jazzercise, or use exercise equipment such as a stationary bike, treadmill, rowing machine, or stair stepper. Begin and end each

20 to 30 minute aerobic session with five minutes of stretching, and strive for five sessions per week. Talk to your doctor about the best training program for you.

- **Strength/resistance training.** Strength training helps you build and maintain muscle strength, as well as helps lower blood sugar levels, maintains bone density, reduces cortisol (a stress hormone) levels, strengthens ligaments and tendons, and increases the production of testosterone (read more about the importance of this hormone in "Balancing Hormones"). Two or three 10-minute sessions of strength or resistance training per week is usually recommended.

Other ways to avoid boredom include exercising with a friend or in a group, exercising to music or while watching TV or a video, and alternating your activities. Having a dog that needs to be exercised is a good way to get you out of the house. Don't have a dog? Offer to walk or jog with a neighbor's dog.

BRAIN EXERCISES

Your brain may not be a muscle, but you can work it like one to help prevent memory loss and other cognitive difficulties associated with aging. As your brain ages, it loses the ability to fight against substances and processes that can harm it, including free radicals and inflammation. Aging brain cells also gradually stop communicating with each other, which affects memory and thought processes. Research shows that B vitamins, including folic acid and niacin, are critical as low levels of this vitamin group are associated with a decline in brain function. Studies also show that a high-fat diet is bad for memory and learning, and that a low-calorie diet helps preserve them.

What You Can Do Now

Along with wise dietary choices, you can keep your brain cells in shape by challenging them daily: do crossword and word puzzles, study a new language or take a class in something that challenges you intellectually, join a book discussion group, volunteer for a cause you believe in, help teach illiterate children to read, attend lectures offered in your community, read a variety of newspapers and magazines from around the world on the Internet, or keep a daily journal.

Although it's not clear exactly how much brain exercises can prevent memory loss and other cognitive difficulties, the results of several large studies provide much promise. In the landmark Nun Study from the 1980s, researchers tested the cognitive ability of 100 nuns who had written their autobiographies fifty years earlier. The scientists found that those who had lower language abilities were at greater risk for Alzheimer's disease. Another study of more than 800 Catholic clergy found that reading newspapers and engaging in other brain-stimulating activities reduced the risk of Alzheimer's disease.

Don't wait. Stimulate those brain cells today!

BALANCING HORMONES

As you age, your body's biochemistry changes, and one of the most significant changes is the decline in the levels of hormones that have a major impact on aging. Specifically, those hormones are the sex hormones—estrogen, progesterone, and testosterone—as well as the mother of all these hormones, DHEA, and a few others, including melatonin, thyroid, and growth hormone.

One of the primary roles of hormones is to transmit messages to the body's cells so they can perform their various functions. Hormone levels begin to decline when people are in their twenties, which means the amount of information that is shared among the cells declines as well. Because hormone levels typically fall slowly, the impact of their decline often isn't felt until people reach their forties or fifties. That's also about the time that women experience another hormonal change—menopause—and men also have a decline in sex hormone production, known as andropause. All of these hormonal changes taken together are associated with symptoms of aging and also increase your chances of developing disease and infection.

Anti-aging medicine promotes hormone balancing using bio-identical hormone therapy as a way to fight aging. The concept is simple: take hormone supplements that are similar to the ones your body produces—not artificial or synthetic hormones—as a means to restore and maintain your levels to where they were when you were in your twenties. Achieving healthy levels and balance of hormones slows the aging process and promotes health and well-being. Generally, hormone balancing offers the following benefits.

- Helps prevent bone loss and osteoporosis.
- Promotes muscle strength and tone.
- Enhances heart functioning.
- Helps maintain a healthy immune system.
- Improves the texture, tone, and elasticity of the skin.
- Improves sexual function and desire.
- Helps maintain mental functioning.
- Promotes tissue repair and regeneration.
- Improves mood and emotional stability.
- Helps keep blood pressure and cholesterol levels down.

What You Can Do Now

Hormone balancing is not an approach you should take on your own: you will need tests to determine your hormone levels and a professional to customize your hormone restoration program. Although most of the hormones are available over the counter, a few require a prescription (testosterone, thyroid) from your physician. A physician should also reevaluate your hormone levels yearly and make any dose adjustments as needed.

STRESS MANAGEMENT

What makes some people go to pieces when there's a two-hour traffic jam and other people take it in stride? A key element is how people decide to manage the stress, and not the fact that a stressful situation has occurred.

Your emotions and thoughts have a significant impact on your health. Stress weakens the immune system, depletes the body of nutrients, disrupts digestion, and causes organs to overwork, increasing the risk for illness and disease. Thus you may eat a nutritious diet, but if you do not manage stress in a healthy way, your body will not benefit from those positive foods. Generally, people who have learned how to manage stressful situations in a healthy way are rewarded with better overall health.

Effective stress management can and should be enjoyable, and there are many techniques you can try and incorporate into your lifestyle to help you better manage stress. Don't limit yourself to just one approach! Exercise is certainly a stress reducer, and so are meditation, tai chi, yoga, playing or listening to music, writing poetry or journaling, or watching humorous movies.

Of course, potentially stress-reducing activities alone won't help you if your attitude is negative. Nurture a positive mental attitude about life and situations as they come. It may sound simplistic, but the truth is that a simple approach is often the one that works, with practice. Only you can decide: is the glass half full or half empty? When you get up in the morning, will you look for the positive in every situation—or the negative?

CHAPTER 2

FROM MARKET TO MEALS

So far we've given you a good idea of the types of foods that offer the best defense against aging and some of the other lifestyle factors that have a direct or indirect impact on those food choices. But if you want to get the most from the food you choose for yourself and your family, you need to know how to select, store, and prepare them. Certain fruits and vegetables, for example, quickly lose their nutritional value if they are stored incorrectly. Some foods, depending on how they are prepared, can accelerate the aging process. For example, deep frying nutrient-rich red onions is far from the best way to enjoy these important vegetables. Meats, poultry, and fish must be handled, stored, and prepared in specific ways to ensure you and your family remain free of food-borne illnesses. It's also important for you to understand how to read nutrition labels and ingredient panels on packaged foods so you can make the best food choices.

All this information and more is discussed in this chapter. Our hope is that you will take the guidelines offered in these pages and use them along with the information provided in the nutrition counter at the back of this book.

GO NATURAL

So far we've discussed many different foods that fight aging—foods that provide essential vitamins, antioxidants, fiber, calcium, quality protein, and good fats. But if you *really* want to reap the most benefits from these anti-aging food choices, you need to think clean—no pesticides, herbicides, hormones, antibiotics, artificial colorings, flavorings, or preservatives. On the surface that may sound like a big order, but if you take it one day at a time, even one food item at a time, before you know it you'll dramatically reduce the amount of damaging toxins you consume through food and beverages.

Experts continue to debate about the benefits of eating organic food. Many studies show, for example, that produce grown under organic conditions have higher levels of nutrients than those grown conventionally. Not every study shows the same degree of benefit, nor that all nutrients are elevated. One recent study of organic and conventional tomatoes, for example, found that organic tomatoes had higher levels of vitamin C, carotenoids, and polyphenols, but when the tomatoes were made into puree, the carotenoid levels were similar between the organic and conventional tomatoes.

A review of 41 published studies in which the nutritional values of organically grown fruits, vegetables, and grains were compared with conventionally grown items found that overall, organic crops had 27% more vitamin C, 21% more iron, 29% more magnesium, and 14% more phosphorus. The review also stated that organic products had 15% fewer nitrates than their conventional counterparts.

Further proof comes from a study conducted by the Organic Materials Review Institute and Consumers Union, which used data from the US Department of Agriculture. The researchers found that 73% of conventionally grown foods sampled had pesticide residue compared with only 23% of organically grown samples of the same crops.

What Is Organic?

According to the US Department of Agriculture's National Organic Program, "organic food is produced by farmers who emphasize the use of renewable resources and the conservation of soil and water to enhance environmental quality. . . . Organic meat, poultry, eggs, and dairy products come from animals that are given no antibiotics or growth hormones." To meet the requirements to be certified organic, foods must be produced without using most conventional pesticides and fertilizers made with synthetic ingredients or sewage sludge. Ionizing radiation and bioengineering are also prohibited. A certified inspector checks organic farms to ensure the food is grown to meet USDA organic standards, and all companies that handle organic food before it reaches the marketplace must be certified as well.

Organic labeling comes in three forms. The name of the certifying agent must appear on all packages:

- **"100% Organic":** must contain 100% organically produced ingredients, not counting added water and salt.
- **"Organic":** must contain at least 95% organically produced ingredients, not counting added water and salt. Must not contain sulfites. May contain up to 5% non-organically produced agricultural ingredients.
- **"Made with Organic Ingredients":** must contain at least 70% organically produced ingredients, not counting added water and salt. Must not contain sulfites. May contain up to 30% non-organically produced agricultural ingredients.

CHOOSE AND USE HEALTHY FATS AND OILS

In Chapter 1 we looked at good fats and bad fats and identified what some of those fats are and the health impacts—both beneficial and damaging—of each type of fat. We also suggested some general ways you can reduce the amount of bad fat and include more healthy fats in your diet.

Now it's time to discuss more specific tips you can use when you go to the supermarket and in your kitchen.

- When choosing oils for cooking and as a condiment, look for cold-pressed oils. These oils are healthier than conventionally produced oils, which are heated, treated with solvents, and bleached. These processes introduce toxins into the oil and also remove much of its nutritional value. Cold-pressed oils are not heated or treated, and so retain their nutritional value. They also contain a higher level of the important antioxidant vitamin E.

- Oils and fat can turn rancid very quickly if they are not stored properly. Rancid fats not only taste terrible, they are carcinogenic as well and have been linked with atherosclerosis and heart disease. The higher the percentage of polyunsaturated fat in an oil, the faster it will go rancid (see chart). To help prevent your oil from going rancid, you should: (1) Refrigerate oil once you open it. Unopened cooking oils have a shelf life of about one year. Unopened oils can be kept unrefrigerated in a cool, dark place. (2) Keep oil in a glass or metal container. If you buy it in a plastic bottle, transfer it to a more suitable container. (3) Buy only as much oil as you think you'll use within a few months' time. (4) Refrigerated oil may turn cloudy, but it will return to normal, unharmed, once it reaches room temperature.

- Avoid use of solid hydrogenated shortening (e.g., Crisco, among others).
- Not all oils are best for every use. Those best as a condiment are olive, hazelnut, sweet almond, sesame, canola, and soy. The first four are also suitable for baking and stir-fry.
- Margarine and vegetable oil spreads. By law, margarine must contains at least 80% fat. Vegetable oil spreads may be reduced-fat, reduced-calorie, or diet (these contain no more than 60% oil); light or lower-fat (contain no more than 40% oil); or fat-free (contain less than 0.5 gram of fat per serving). Both margarines and spreads are made from vegetable oils, with the healthiest ones (those highest in monounsaturated fat and lowest in saturated fat) being olive oil, flaxseed oil, hempseed oil, and canola oil.

FAT CONTENT OF OILS

Oil	Mono.	Poly.	Sat.
Olive	77%	9%	14%
Avocado	74%	14%	12%
Almond	73%	18%	9%
Apricot	63%	31%	6%
Canola	62%	31%	7%
Peanut	48%	34%	18%
Sesame	42%	43%	15%
Corn	25%	62%	20%

FAT CONTENT OF OILS

Oil	Mono.	Poly.	Sat.
Soybean	24%	61%	15%
Sunflower	20%	69%	11%
Cottonseed	19%	54%	27%
Safflower	13%	78%	9%

FRUITS AND VEGETABLES

It's no secret that fruits and vegetables are a criti-
cally important part of an anti-aging diet; after all,
they are a super source of age-defying antioxidants,
fiber, and other nutrients; they are low in fat and sodium, and they have no cholesterol. Add to this list
the fact that there are dozens and dozens of choices
from which to choose, and you can't go wrong.

Or can you? The benefits of eating fruits and
vegetables are greatly diminished or eliminated if
the produce isn't selected or stored properly, or if
it is prepared in unhealthy ways. Although every
fruit and vegetable has its own unique characteristics, here are some general guidelines for pur-
chasing, handling, and eating produce so you can
enjoy and reap the health rewards they have to
offer.

- Wash all produce, whether conventionally or
  organically grown, just before serving or cooking, not before you store them. Cool water is all
  that's necessary; commercial produce washes
  offer little or no advantage over plain water.

- Check the PLU stickers on your produce. Conventionally grown produce has a four-digit number (e.g., 1234); organically grown, five digits prefaced by the number 9 (e.g., 91234); and genetically modified produce, five digits prefaced by the number 8 (e.g., 81234).
- Discard the outer leaves of leafy vegetables because pesticide residues tend to accumulate there.
- Use a produce brush to clean firm produce (e.g., carrots, potatoes, turnips).
- Immediately refrigerate any produce that you cut and do not plan to eat right away, as bacteria grow very quickly on cut fruits and vegetables.
- Wash fruits and vegetables that you peel (e.g., melons, oranges, pineapples) because when you cut them, your knife transfers contaminants from the peel into the pulp.
- Do not buy or use produce that is moldy, badly bruised, shriveled, or slimy. Minor blemishes are usually safe; in fact, organic produce sometimes has minor blemishes because it is not colored, waxed, or has not undergone attempts to make it look "perfect."
- Do not store fruits and greens together, because fruits give off ethylene gas, which causes greens to decay.
- Always cook dehydrated vegetables thoroughly, as they are susceptible to contamination by various microorganisms and can cause foodborne illness.

- To freeze most vegetables, steam blanch them (see blanching guidelines at http://www.ext.colo state.edu/PUBS/FOODNUT/09330.pdf). Blanching stops the enzymes from breaking down the nutrients in the vegetables. Cool and then store blanched vegetables in freezer bags or containers.

HOW TO READ FOOD LABELS

Nutrition Facts labels and other labeling on food packages can provide much important information when choosing age-defying foods, but they can also be confusing. So we try to sort it out for you.

Nutrition Facts Labels

Nutrition Facts labels are required for most foods (except meat and poultry) and have standardized categories, which we explain here.

- Serving Size and Servings Per Container: If the serving size is 1 cup and there are 2 servings per container, then the package contains 2 cups. If you eat two servings rather than one, you must remember to double the values of the calories, nutrients, and % daily value figures below this line on the label.
- Calories and Calories from Fat: these values are per serving.
- % Daily Value: These percentages are based on the Daily Value recommendations for important

nutrients, based on a 2,000 calorie daily diet. You may eat fewer or more than 2,000 calories daily, but you can still use this figure as a reference point. The % DV helps you determine if a serving of a food is low or high in a specific nutrient. Each nutrient is based on 100% of the daily requirements for that nutrient. A value of 5% or less is considered low; 20% or more is considered high.

- Total Fat, Saturated Fat, Trans Fat, Sodium, and Cholesterol: These substances are ones you want to limit because they are associated with accelerated aging and disease. Therefore, preferred foods contain a % DV of 5% or less.

- Sugars: No % DV has been established for sugars. The sugars listed on Nutrition Facts labels include naturally occurring sugars (e.g., those in fruit and milk) and added sugars. Added sugars will appear on the ingredient portion of the label and may be listed as sugar, corn syrup, high-fructose corn syrup, maltose, dextrose, sucrose, honey, fruit juice concentrate, and maple syrup.

- Dietary Fiber, Vitamin A, Vitamin C, Calcium, Iron: These nutrients are among those you want to see in the high range: % DV of 20% or more.

- Protein: Manufacturers must give a % DV only if the food claims to be high in protein or if the food is meant for infants and children younger than 4 years old.

- "Percent Daily Values" Footnote: The following statement must appear on all Nutrition

Facts labels. "Percent Daily Values are based on a 2,000 calorie diet. Your Daily Values may be higher or lower depending on your calorie needs." The remaining information does not need to appear if the package is too small. When the information does appear, it is the same on all products, because it is general dietary advice for all Americans.

Light, Low, Free, Lean: What's It All Mean?

The Food and Drug Administration (FDA) has established definitions and guidelines for terms that can appear on food packaging. Here's a sample.

- **Free:** the product contains no amount of, or only a trivial or "physiologically inconsequential" amount of one or more of these substances: fat, saturated fat, cholesterol, sodium, sugars, and calories.
- **Low fat:** the product contains 3 grams of fat or less per serving.
- **Low saturated fat:** 1 g or less per serving.
- **Low sodium:** 140 mg or less per serving.
- **Very low sodium:** 35 mg or less per serving.
- **Low cholesterol:** 20 mg or less and 2 g or less of saturated fat per serving.
- **Low calorie:** 40 calories or less per serving.
- **Lean and extra lean:** when describing meat, poultry, seafood, and game, "lean" means it contains less than 10 g of fat, 4.5 g or less saturated fat, and less than 95 mg cholesterol per

serving and per 100 g. "Extra lean" means it contains less than 5 g fat, less than 2 g saturated fat, and less than 95 mg cholesterol per serving and per 100 g.

- **High:** means the food contains 20% or more of the Daily Value for a specific nutrient.
- **Good Source:** means that one serving of the product contains 10 to 19 percent of the Daily Value for a specific nutrient.
- **Light:** can mean one of three things: (1) the food contains one-third fewer calories or half the fat of the reference food. If the food provides 50% or more of its calories from fat, the reduction must be 50% of the fat. (2) The sodium content of a low-calorie, low-fat food has been reduced by 50%. (3) The term describes color, texture, or another property of the food, but the label must explain the term, such as "light brown sugar."
- **Fresh:** the FDA defines this term when it is used for foods that are raw or unprocessed. Thus "fresh" can be used only on raw foods, ones that have never been frozen or heated, and contain no preservatives. "Fresh frozen," "frozen fresh," and "freshly frozen" can be used for foods that were rapidly frozen while still fresh.

EGG SAFETY

Eggs are a good source of protein, low in fat (if you limit yourself to the whites), and relatively inexpensive, so it is often on an anti-aging menu. Proper handling and preparation are critical, however, especially since it is estimated that 1 out of every 10,000 eggs (about 4.5 million eggs per year) are infected with *Salmonella enteritidis*, which causes food poisoning. Because contaminated eggs do not look or smell any different than non-contaminated eggs, it isn't possible to know if any of the eggs you purchase are affected.

The notion that "free-range" eggs are healthier and produced in less cruel conditions than conventional eggs is largely untrue. In most cases, free-range egg producers keep their hens uncaged but confined to overly crowded facilities that have very limited access to the outdoors, or they are confined to cages that are larger than those used to hold conventionally raised hens. There are no government laws that regulate the meaning of "free-range," so unless you personally see the conditions under which your eggs are produced, you cannot be sure that the higher prices you pay for free-range eggs are supporting a healthier product produced in less cruel conditions.

Choosing and Preparing Eggs

- If possible, buy your eggs from local producers (with a facility that you can visit). They may sell from their farm or at a farmers' market.
- Purchase eggs that are refrigerated at 40°F or lower.

- Do not purchase eggs that are cracked.
- When you get the eggs home, immediately place them in the coldest part of the refrigerator (in the rear), not on the door.
- If you accidentally crack an egg before you are ready to use it, break the egg into a clean container, cover it tightly, and refrigerate it. Use it within 2 days.
- Cook eggs until the yolks and whites are firm. Do not eat lightly poached or soft-boiled eggs.
- Never eat raw eggs or foods that contain raw eggs (e.g., eggnog, Hollandaise sauce).
- Do not leave eggs unrefrigerated for longer than two hours.

MEAT, POULTRY, AND FISH

Proper handling and preparation of meats, fish, and poultry are critical because the potential for contamination and food poisoning is high. Contamination can occur at several levels. According to the Humane Farming Association, only a small percentage of the meat processed in U.S. slaughterhouses is tested for toxins (e.g., dioxins, PCBs, pesticides) that get into the meat supply either through the animals' feed and/or water, or through direct means (injections of antibiotics, hormones). Contamination or compromise of meat, poultry, and fish can also occur anywhere during processing, from packing and shipping to the market and finally your kitchen. Therefore, consider these important guidelines.

Meat and Poultry

- Buy organically produced meat and poultry. Compared with conventionally produced items, they expose you to significantly fewer age-accelerating and disease-causing substances.
- Cook meat and poultry thoroughly and always check the temperature with a meat thermometer. Different meats and cuts have different safe temperatures, so be sure to check the cooking instructions. (See www.foodsafety. gov/~fsg/fs-cook.html for safe cooking temperatures.) Do not depend on the color of the meat to determine if it has been cooked adequately.
- Thaw frozen meat in the refrigerator, which can take eight or more hours. If you need to defrost it more quickly, place it in a sealed plastic bag and immerse the bag in a pot of cold water for an hour.
- Wash your hands with soap and hot water before and after handling raw meat.
- Marinate meat and poultry in the refrigerator. Once the food has been marinated, discard the marinade because raw juice from the meat or poultry may contain bacteria.
- Do not eat the organs (e.g., brains, livers, kid-

neys) of livestock, because poisons accumulate in them.

Fish

- Buy only fresh fish and seafood that is refrigerated or frozen.
- Frozen fish should be in a package that is transparent so you can see sign of crystals or frost. If you do, the fish has been thawed and refrozen.
- Refrigerate or freeze fish immediately when you bring it home. You should also transport it in an ice chest in the car.
- Do not buy shellfish that has a strong "fishy" smell, because it may be spoiled.
- Rinse and rewrap fish when you get it home. Place it on paper towels, put it in a tightly covered container, and place it in the coldest part of the refrigerator.
- Throw away any fat drippings from boiled or poached fish, as toxins accumulate in the fat.
- Before cooking fish, remove skin and fatty tissue from the sides, belly, and along the top of the back. This is where many toxins accumulate. Mercury, however, accumulates mainly in the muscle, so it can't be removed. To minimize your exposure to mercury, choose fish that typically contain low levels of mercury (e.g., salmon, herring, sardines, anchovies, tilapia). The U.S.

FDA maintains a website that lists mercury levels in fish and seafood at www.cfsan.fda.gov/~frf/sea-mehg.html.

- Cook fish and seafood until the internal temperature is at least 145°F; for stuffed fish, at least 165°F. (See www.foodsafety.gov/~fsg/fs-cook.html for safe cooking temperatures.)

CHAPTER 3

10-STEP
ANTI-AGING DIET

We have loaded you up with lots of important information about how food and optimal food choices and preparation can help you fight aging. Now we're going to pull it all together into a manageable 10-Step Anti-Aging Diet Plan that's based on recommendations from leading health experts and health organizations, including the American Heart Association and the American Diabetes Association.

STEP 1: WATCH YOUR FATS

As a general guideline, you should hold your total fat intake to 25 to 30 percent of calories, and no more than 10 percent of total caloric intake should be from "bad" fats—saturated and trans fats. Trans fat should be held to 3% or less. The remaining 15 to 20 percent of total calories that are reserved for fat intake should come from "good" fats—monounsaturated and omega-3 fatty acids.

Watching your fats is easy if you follow a few simple guidelines.

- If you eat dairy products, choose no-fat and low-fat varieties.
- When considering protein foods, choose fish, lean cuts of meat, egg whites, and skinless poultry. Plant-based protein is generally much lower in fat than animal foods. Choose dried beans, lentils, tempeh, peas, or tofu in place of meat.
- Use olive oil (extra virgin if you can), which is especially rich in monounsaturated fat and antioxidants, both of which protect against aging, coronary heart disease, and cancer. Use it for stir-fry or as a salad dressing. Second best choices are flaxseed, canola, and peanut oils.
- Avoid trans fats: read ingredient labels and look for the words "hydrogenated" or "partially hydrogenated" oil or margarine. Also look at the nutrition label for the amount of trans fat in a product. Even if the nutrition label says zero trans fat per serving, food manufacturers are allowed to say zero if one serving contains less than 0.5 grams of trans fat.

STEP 2: BE NUTS ABOUT NUTS

You should be nuts about nuts, and here's why. Several very large studies that included tens of thousands of participants from the Nurses' Health Study, the Physicians' Health Study, and others, found that the risk of coronary heart disease is 37 percent lower among people who eat nuts more than four times per week compared with those who never or seldom eat nuts. Experts believe the reason is that most nuts are high in monounsaturated fats, which help lower low-density lipoprotein cholesterol. Nuts are a rich source of B vitamins, which are good for the heart and brain. They also contain healthy fats, which also benefit the heart and circulation, as well as the collagen and elastin in the skin, helping it maintain elasticity and resiliency.

Because nuts are high in calories, small portions are advised. The best way to enjoy the flavor and benefits of nuts is to eat them as a snack in place of chips or another "junk" food, or sprinkle them on cereal, salad, or in stir-fry.

STEP 3: ENJOY AN ABUNDANCE OF ANTIOXIDANTS

We've mentioned the impact that free radicals have on aging, so you need lots of antioxidants to fight off these nasty damaging molecules. The accumulated harm to cells, tissues, and organs caused by free radicals is a key contributor to aging and many diseases associated with growing older. Great sources of antioxidants are fresh fruits and vegetables, which are generally rich in vitamins, minerals, and phytonutrients. Phytonutrients ("phyto" means "plant") are chemicals that give fruits and vegetables their color. Carotenoids, flavonoids, indoles, and catechins are just a few of the many different types of phytonutrients.

Phytonutrients and other antioxidants are especially helpful in the fight against aging and in promoting wellness. Aim to eat one or more servings daily from each of the following groups of fruits and vegetables, which are rich in phytonutrients.

- **Green:** dark green, leafy vegetables (romaine lettuce [skip the iceberg!], spinach, kale, mustard greens, swiss chard), green peppers, broccoli, peas, avocado, celery.
- **Yellow/orange:** carrots, yellow peppers, apricots, peaches, pineapple, oranges, yellow squash, pumpkin, yams and sweet potatoes, acorn squash, spaghetti squash.
- **Red:** red peppers, tomatoes, blood oranges, cherries, cranberries, strawberries, red leaf lettuce, red apples.
- **Blue/purple:** blueberries, eggplant, raisins, plums, blackberries, purple cabbage.
- **White:** cauliflower, mushrooms, turnips, apple juice, parsnips, white onions, white peaches, garlic.

STEP 4: STOP INFLAMMATION
WITH EVERY MEAL

Inflammation doesn't just affect the joints and cause arthritis; it can occur anywhere along the miles of blood vessels in the body. In fact, recent research shows that chronic inflammation of the blood vessels is an important factor in aging and age-related diseases, including heart disease, stroke, diabetes, cancer, and Alzheimer's disease. A major contributor to that inflammation is the Standard American Diet (SAD).

That means you can begin to fight inflammation right now by making some dietary changes. You can also learn to what extent your blood vessels are affected by inflammation by asking your doctor to order a C-reactive protein test. The higher your value on this simple blood test, the greater your level of inflammation and your risk for these diseases.

You can slow down the aging process and reduce your risk for disease when you choose foods that fight, reduce, or prevent inflammation. Here are some tips.

- **Be sugar smart.** Foods that raise blood glucose levels also promote inflammation. Choose complex carbohydrate foods—whole grains, beans, lentils, fruits and vegetables, nuts and seeds—and avoid or limit your intake of sugar and sugary foods, highly processed cereals and baked goods, white rice, white potatoes, white bread, and high fructose corn syrup (found in many processed foods).

- **Watch your protein.** A high-protein diet can boost blood vessel inflammation, as high as 62% according to one study, and worsen coronary artery disease as well. Keep your protein intake to about 20 percent of your total caloric intake per day.

- **Eat cold-water fatty fish.** Fish such as salmon, herring, sardines, and tuna contain a good source of omega-3 fatty acids, which suppress the substances that cause inflammation in the body. Include these fish two or three times a week in your diet.

- **Include powerhouse anti-inflammatory foods daily.** Many foods have been identified as possessing anti-inflammatory powers. Make sure to include as many of them as you can in your daily diet. They are as follows: members of the *Allium* family—onions, garlic (which also helps reduce cholesterol and blood pressure), chives, shallots; barley; beans and lentils; buckwheat; blueberries; yogurt and kefir (a fermented milk beverage); curry powder; acai fruit.

- **Turn down the heat.** Foods that are prepared using high cooking temperatures contain advanced glycation end products, or AGEs, which trigger inflammation. When preparing meats, poultry, fish, and vegetables, healthy cooking techniques include steaming, poaching, boiling, slow-cooking (in a crockpot), and stir-frying. Limit the amounts of food that you fry, broil, grill, or bake.

STEP 5: MAKE FRIENDS WITH FIBER

It's not hard to make friends with fiber if you follow steps 3 and 4, because they include plenty of fiber-rich foods. The Institutes of Medicine recommend the following daily fiber intake (soluble and insoluble) for adults: for men 19 to 50 years, 38 grams per day; older than 50 years, 30 grams. For women 19 to 50 years, 25 grams per day; older than 50 years, 21 grams. You can use the nutrition counter in the back of the book to help you identify how much fiber you are getting now and which foods can help you meet your goals if you fall short, as most Americans do.

The best sources of fiber are whole grains, legumes, beans, fruits and vegetables (with skins on when possible), nuts and seeds, and high-fiber cereals. If you need to increase your fiber intake, consider the following.

- Add high-fiber foods gradually. If you eat 8 to 10 grams per day now, for example, increase to 13 to 15 grams for a few days, then add another 5 grams for several more days, until you reach your goal. Too rapid an increase may cause stomach upset, cramps, or bloating.

- Increase your water intake as you increase your fiber to help your body adjust to the change and to prevent constipation.

STEP 6: HYDRATE YOUR BODY

Pure water is essential for hydration of the skin and muscles and to promote healthy circulation and organ system functioning, especially the gastrointestinal system. Keeping yourself properly hydrated can also significantly reduce your chances of getting cancer. Studies have shown that women who drank more water (eight glasses or more daily) had less than 50% the risk of developing colon cancer and 80% less chance of developing bladder cancer than women who drank less.

The general consensus is to drink 8 to 10 eight-ounce glasses of water per day, and this is a good starting point. However, everyone's needs are different. The temperature of your environment, your current state of health, how much exercise you do, whether you are pregnant or breastfeeding, and how much water you get from your food (20% is the average) are all factors to consider when deciding how much water you need to consume daily.

You are probably drinking enough fluid if you eliminate between 32 and 64 ounces of colorless or slightly yellow urine daily. Darker urine usually indicates that you need to increase your water intake. Do not wait until you are thirsty to drink water: by that time, you may already be slightly dehydrated. The ability to identify dehydration becomes more difficult with age because the body is less able to send the brain signals that it is thirsty. To help ensure you are getting enough water:

- Drink one glass of water before each meal and one between meals. These should be taken slowly, not gulped down.
- Drink water before, during, and after you exercise.
- Brighten your water with a squeeze of lemon or lime.
- If you increase the amount of fiber in your diet, you will likely need to add 1 or 2 more eight-ounce glasses of water daily.
- Substitute a glass of sparkling water for alcohol at social events.

STEP 7: OPTIMIZE YOUR PROTEIN INTAKE

Protein deficiency is one dietary problem most Americans do *not* have, but getting too much protein—and suboptimal protein—is. To this fact add another one: as you age your ability to create, transport, and break down proteins decreases. The combined result is a loss of muscle tone, the appearance of wrinkles, loss and graying of hair, less energy, joint stiffness, and a host of other difficulties. Excess protein can be converted into fat, and it also places stress on the liver and kidneys as these organs try to rid the body of unwanted by-products of metabolism. Too much protein can also cause dehydration and your kidneys to excrete calcium in urine, which increases your risk for osteoporosis.

To optimize the anti-aging power of your protein intake, first calculate your protein needs: the RDA for protein for adults is 0.36 grams of protein per pound of body weight per day. Therefore, if you weigh 150 pounds, your protein requirement is $150 \times 0.36 = 54$ grams. Remember, 0.36 g/lb is an average.

- Choose lean cuts of meat from animals that were organically raised.
- Avoid processed meats, including hot dogs, smoked meats, bacon, sausages, ham, and cold cuts. These foods are usually high in saturated fat, sodium, and artificial colorings, flavorings, and preservatives, including cancer-causing nitrates and nitrites.
- Include plant-based protein in your diet. Beans, legumes, veggie burgers, tempeh, and soy-based "meats" often have just as much protein, if not more, than a comparable amount of animal protein, and without the saturated fat (soybeans do contain some fat).
- Eat protein with carbohydrates. (A turkey sandwich on whole-grain bread or tofu with brown rice are examples of this nutrient combination.) Protein takes longer to digest than carbs, so it

slows down the release of glucose into your bloodstream. The result is that you will feel more energetic.

• Eggs and egg whites are a good source of protein. Some brands are from animals that have been fed fortified feed that enhances the omega-3 fatty acid content of the eggs.

STEP 8: COOK THE ANTI-AGING WAY

It's not always what you eat but how you prepare it that can subtract years from your life. That's why you need to prepare your food in ways that do not promote the formation of advanced glycation end products (AGEs), those nasty substances that accelerate aging, cause inflammation, and contribute to dozens of diseases and illnesses. Healthy cooking methods include poaching, boiling, stir-frying, slow-cooking (crockpot), and steaming; avoid baking, grilling, broiling, and microwaving. The same holds true for meals you order at restaurants.

STEP 9: STRIVE TO BE TOXIN FREE

You are surrounded by substances that cause and contribute to aging and disease, and that includes the food and beverages you consume every day. Fortunately there are ways you can avoid or minimize their harmful effects.

- Avoid sugar and sugary foods. If you don't think something that tastes so good and sweet could be so bad, think again. Sugar and refined carbohydrates cause inflammation, especially of the blood vessels; are associated with insulin resistance, diabetes, and ultimately the complications associated with diabetes; promote the formation of AGEs; hinder the absorption of calcium, which contributes to the development of osteoporosis; suppresses the release of growth hormone, which is responsible for the repair and regeneration of cells and tissues and maintaining bone strength, brain function, and muscle tone; and causes or contributes to dozens of other health problems. And not all sugars are created equally: fructose, for example, promotes glycation at a rate nearly seven times that of glucose. Fructose is found naturally in unrefined foods such as fruits and vegetables, but processed foods often contain added fructose.
- Choose organic fruits and vegetables to help avoid exposure to pesticides, herbicides, and other agricultural poisons.
- Choose hormone-free meats, poultry, dairy, and eggs. Better yet, regularly substitute plant-based protein foods for animal-based ones, as they are naturally hormone-free.
- Avoid highly processed foods, especially processed meats such as bologna, sausage, smoked

meats, and hot dogs, which often contain
cancer-causing nitrates and nitrites.

• Avoid or seriously limit consumption of refined, processed foods, as they contain artificial flavorings, colorings, and preservatives.

• Eat fish that is as mercury-free as possible. All
fish and seafood contain at least a small amount
of mercury and/or other toxins, especially large
fish because they usually live longer and eat
other fish that are contaminated. Those with
a minimal amount of toxins generally include
sardines, herring, cod, pollock, salmon, and
anchovies.

STEP 10: DRINK GREEN TEA

Unlike black and oolong tea, green tea is not fermented, so its active ingredients are not changed.
Some of those ingredients include polyphenols, potent antioxidants that appear to help protect against
various cancers. Green tea is also credited with
helping regulate blood glucose levels, lowering cholesterol levels, and helping promote weight loss. The
polyphenols in green tea are also believed to stimulate the production of immune system cells and to
directly inhibit glycation. Studies in both humans
and animals suggest that green tea may reduce the
risk of cardiovascular disease, promote oral health,
lower blood pressure, protect the nervous system,
and have antibacterial and antiviral properties.

To reap the anti-aging benefits of green tea, drink at least three cups daily. Green tea does contain some caffeine, but at a much lower level than in coffee: an eight-ounce cup of green tea has about 20 to 30 mg of caffeine, compared with about 100 mg in a cup of coffee. Decaffeinated green tea is also available.

CHAPTER 4

A SAMPLE ANTI-AGING MENU

To help you get started on your anti-aging eating plan, here is a three-day menu complete with recipes. The menu and recipes incorporate the information and guidelines that appear in chapters 1 through 3. Menu items that have a recipe are in italics. All of the recipes follow the sample menu plan.

Day 1

BREAKFAST
Oat bran with walnuts and raisins
½ grapefruit
1 cup green tea

MID-MORNING SNACK
1 cup vegetable juice with lemon

LUNCH
  Favorite Bean Chili
  Whole-grain crackers
  Fresh pear, apple, or banana
  Seltzer water w/lemon

MID-AFTERNOON SNACK
  8 ounces 2% milk or soy milk

DINNER
  Poached Salmon
  Veggie Rice Casserole
  Avocado Salad (red leaf lettuce, avocado, red
  pepper, tomato, olive oil, and vinegar)
  $\frac{1}{2}$ cup blueberries

Day 2

BREAKFAST
  Scrambled Delight
  $\frac{1}{2}$ whole-grain bagel
  1 cup green tea

MID-MORNING SNACK
  1 banana or $\frac{1}{4}$ cantaloupe

LUNCH
  Red, Green, and Bean Salad
  Whole-grain rye crackers
  1 cup low-fat milk or soy milk

MID-AFTERNOON SNACK
　8-ounce container low-fat plain yogurt with ¼
　cup blueberries or strawberries and 1 tbs wheat
　germ

DINNER
　Festive Fettuccine
　Brussels Sprouts in Orange Sauce
　1 cup green tea

Day 3

BREAKFAST
　Sunrise Quinoa with fresh fruit
　1 slice whole-grain bread with all-fruit jelly
　1 cup green tea

MID-MORNING SNACK
　Mango Smoothie

LUNCH
　Split Pea and Veggie Stew
　½ whole-wheat pita
　Iced herbal tea

MID-AFTERNOON SNACK
　Raw vegetables with *Eggplant dip*

DINNER
　Chicken, Veggie, and Cashew Stir-fry
　Brown rice

RECIPES FOR DAY 1

OAT BRAN WITH WALNUTS AND RAISINS

1 serving
   ⅓ cup oat bran
   ½ cup apple juice
   ½ cup low-fat soy milk
   1 tbs wheat germ
   1 tbs raisins
   3 walnut halves, chopped

Combine the bran, juice, milk, and wheat germ in a small saucepan. Heat over low heat until the mixture boils and stir constantly. Cook for 3 minutes. Remove from the heat and cover; let stand 1 minute. Stir in the raisins and walnuts.

FAVORITE BEAN CHILI

Serves 4–6
   *1 cup each chopped onion, diced carrot, diced
      celery*
   1 cup water
   3 cloves garlic, minced
   ½ cup chopped red, green, or yellow pepper
   1½ tbs chili powder
   ½ tsp cayenne
   2 tsp mustard
   2 28-oz cans crushed tomatoes (save the juice)

> **5 cups of cooked beans—your favorites in any**
> **combination—pinto, black, garbanzo, soy,**
> **kidney; lentils are good, too**
> **Salt to taste**

In a large saucepan, simmer the onion in 1 cup water over medium heat for about 2 minutes, then add
the garlic, carrot, celery, pepper, chili powder, tomatoes, and cayenne. Simmer and stir until well
blended, then add the beans. Lower heat and simmer low for 30 minutes. Add the mustard and salt,
stir, and serve.

POACHED SALMON

Serves 1
> **1 salmon fillet**
> **¼ cup white wine**
> **¼ cup water**
> **Several thin slices of red onion and green pepper**
> **Dash of dill**

Put the wine, water, dill, onions, and pepper in a
sauté pan and simmer on medium heat. Place the
fillet in the pan. Cover and cook until done, about
5 minutes depending on the thickness of the fillet.
Do not overcook.

VEGGIE RICE CASSEROLE

Serves 4

> *1 large clove garlic, peeled*
> *Handful of fresh cilantro leaves*
> *½ cup fresh parsley leaves*
> *¼ cup chopped onion*
> *2½ cups vegetable broth*
> *1 cup short grain brown rice*
> *1 green bell pepper, chopped*
> *1 large carrot, shredded*

Place the garlic, cilantro, onion, and ½ cup broth in a food processor and process until finely chopped. In a medium-size pot, bring the remaining broth to a boil and add the chopped mixture. Slowly add the rice, green pepper, and shredded carrot, reduce the heat, cover, and simmer for 35 to 45 minutes or until all the liquid has been absorbed.

Garnish with parsley.

RECIPES FOR DAY 2

SCRAMBLED DELIGHT

Serves 2

> *½ green pepper, chopped*
> *½ red pepper, chopped*
> *½ onion, chopped*
> *½ cup spinach, chopped*
> *Water for steaming*

1 clove garlic, minced
1 tsp extra virgin olive oil
4 eggs
Dash of salt and pepper

In a skillet, steam all the vegetables and garlic in a few tablespoons of water until moderately soft. Add oil to the pan and mix to make sure the vegetables and pan are coated. Whisk the eggs in a bowl and add them to the pan; add salt and pepper and cook until desired consistency is reached.

RED, GREEN, AND BEAN SALAD

Serves 4

1 head romaine or red-leaf lettuce
¾ cup chickpeas
¾ cup black beans
1 cup shredded bok choy
1 cup shredded red cabbage
⅓ cup grated low-fat or non-fat cheddar cheese
1 tsp olive oil
2 tbs lemon juice
1 tbs red wine vinegar (or other vinegar)
½ cup chopped walnuts or pecans

Wash, drain, and tear the lettuce into small pieces. Place in a bowl and add the cabbage, beans and chickpeas, bok choy, and cheese. In a small bowl beat the oil, lemon juice, and vinegar. Pour the

dressing onto the salad, add the nuts, and toss
lightly.

FESTIVE FETTUCCINE

Serves 4

   10 oz whole-grain fettuccine
   2 cloves garlic, minced
   ½ lb cubed firm tofu, or 1 cup shredded cooked
      chicken breast
   1 tbs extra virgin olive oil
   1½ lbs ripe tomatoes, cut into 1-inch pieces
      (you can also use canned chopped tomatoes)
   1 cup fresh basil leaves, packed
   ¼ lb asparagus, cut into one-inch pieces
   1 cup frozen green peas, thawed
   Salt and pepper to taste

Cook the pasta according to package directions.
Drain and reserve ⅓ cup cooking liquid. In a large
skillet, heat the oil, and lightly sauté the garlic, asparagus, and tofu for 1 minute. Add tomatoes and
peas and reserved liquid (and chicken if using
chicken). Cook for 1 minute. Add the cooked pasta
and toss. Remove from heat and add the basil, salt,
and pepper. Serve immediately.

BRUSSELS SPROUTS IN ORANGE SAUCE

Serves 4

1 lb brussels sprouts
1½ tsp cornstarch
¼ cup orange juice
1 orange, peeled and sectioned
¼ cup fresh cilantro, chopped
⅛ cup slivered almonds

Cut a cross into the base of each sprout. Steam the sprouts until tender, about 15 to 20 minutes. In a small saucepan, combine the cornstarch and orange juice. Heat over low heat stirring constantly until thickened. Add the orange sections and cook until bubbly. Pour over the sprouts and serve with cilantro and almond garnish.

RECIPES FOR DAY 3

SUNRISE QUINOA WITH FRESH FRUIT

Serves 4

3 cups cooked quinoa
3 apricots, chopped
1 orange, peeled and sectioned
1 cup seedless red grapes, halved
¼ cup raisins
¼ cup chopped walnuts or pecans

Combine all ingredients except the nuts in a bowl and chill for 1 hour or overnight. Top with nuts before serving.

MANGO SMOOTHIE

1 serving
  1 banana
  1 mango (peeled and pitted)
  8 ounces orange juice

Place all ingredients in a blender or food processor and blend until smooth. Or, you can mash the fruits, place them in a jar with a tight lid, add the juice, and shake vigorously.

SPLIT PEA AND VEGGIE STEW

Serves 4
  1 cup dry green split peas
  3 cups water
  ¼ lb each green beans cut into 1-inch pieces,
    chopped zucchini, and sliced mushrooms
  1 green pepper, chopped
  1 tbs soy sauce
  1 tsp mustard

Place split peas and water in a large pot and bring to a boil; reduce heat, cover, and simmer 1 hour. Steam the vegetables until tender. Combine the cooked split peas and vegetables, stir in soy sauce and mustard, and serve.

EGGPLANT DIP

Makes 1½ cups
   1 large eggplant
   2 cloves garlic, minced
   1 green onion, chopped
   ¼ cup chopped parsley
   1 tbs lemon juice
   10 black olives, pitted and chopped

Peel the eggplant and cut it into quarters. Place the pieces into a steamer and steam until tender, about 10 minutes. When cool, press the liquid out of the eggplant. Place the cooked eggplant and all the remaining ingredients except the olives into a blender and blend until smooth. (If you want a chunky dip, you can hand-mash the ingredients.) Add the chopped olives and chill before serving.

CHICKEN, VEGGIE, AND CASHEW STIR-FRY

Serves 4
   ½ lb chicken breast, poached and cut into
      ⅛-inch wide, 3-inch long strips
   1 tsp extra virgin olive oil
   1 clove garlic, minced
   ½ cup sliced carrots

½ cup sliced onion
½ cup sliced green pepper
1 cup bean sprouts
2 cups zucchini, cut into thin strips
¼ cup cashew pieces
1 tbs soy sauce
1 tbs cornstarch
¼ cup water

Heat oil in a skillet and sauté the garlic for 1 minute. Add the carrots, onion, green pepper, and soy sauce, cover, and stir fry for 3 to 4 minutes. Add zucchini, bean sprouts, and cooked chicken and stir fry for 3 to 4 minutes. Mix cornstarch and water until smooth. Pour it slowly into the chicken and vegetable mixture, stirring constantly. Cook until thickened and the mixture is well coated. Toss in cashew pieces and serve with brown rice.

CHAPTER 5

THE ANTI-AGING NUTRITION COUNTER

*F*oods That Combat Aging is a one-stop guide to common, everyday foods and nutrients that can help you fight the aging process with every meal. In the nutrition counter you'll find information about calories, portion size, total fat, good fats, bad fats, fiber, calcium, sugars, the antioxidants vitamin C and beta-carotene, and the B vitamins. We hope you will use this information to help you make informed, healthy choices as you purchase, prepare, and enjoy your meals.

HOW TO FIND YOUR FOODS

All food items are arranged alphabetically. For example, if you want to find peppers, turn to the nutrition counter and look for "peppers." Under "peppers" you will see that there are several types of peppers, and you can easily compare the nutritional values of each.

Some foods have been placed in categories. One of the food categories is "Frozen Dinners and Entrees." Dinners represent entire meals, which generally are packaged to include an entrée (e.g., lasagna, meatloaf, fish fillet), a side vegetable, and a dessert. An *entrée* is packaged to contain the main food item only (e.g., pasta, chicken breast, fish fillet).

No nutrition counter would be complete without a fast food category, and ours lists foods alphabetically for many of the most popular fast food establishments in the United States. You already know that you need to limit or avoid most fast foods and other treats such as cookies, candies, and doughnuts and that you should look for nutritious alternatives instead. That's why we have included healthier versions of these treats whenever possible. The counter makes it easy for you to compare the helpful and harmful nutrients in similar foods so you can make an informed choice.

NOTE: The DRI (Daily Recommended Intake) is an expansion of the RDA (Recommended Daily Allowance) designation, which is being phased out. It's important to understand that RDA and DRI values are based on the minimum amount needed by healthy individuals to maintain an adequate amount of the given nutrient in the body. These values are not sufficient for people who are already deficient in any one or more nutrients and/or anyone who has a medical condition or is exposed to conditions that make higher levels of the nutrient desirable. Basically, the DRIs and RDAs are too low for nearly everyone, and especially if you want to fight aging, so they should be used as a guideline only.

HOW TO IDENTIFY ANTI-AGING NUTRIENTS

Each of the food entries in the nutrition counter has information in the following categories: food name, portion size, calories, total fat, good fats, bad fats, fiber, sugar, beta-carotene, calcium, vitamin C, and B vitamins. Let's look at each of these categories more closely.

Portion Size

This is the standard amount of food suggested by the U.S. Department of Agriculture and the food industry. Always check the serving size: it may be smaller or larger than you think.

Calories

This is the amount of energy provided by one serving of a food or beverage. You can use this value to help you plan your meals if you are trying to lose weight or restrict your total daily caloric intake.

Total Fat

The figure in the total fat category is the sum of saturated, monounsaturated, polyunsaturated, and trans fats. We break down these four types of fat into two subcategories (bad fats and good fats) in other columns.

Overall, your daily fat intake should be 20 to 25 percent of your total daily calories. Based on a 2,000-calorie-per-day diet, that translates as 2,000 calories × 20% (or 25%) = 400 (or 500) ÷ 9 (calories per gram of fat) = 44 (or 50) grams, which = 396 (or 450) calories. You can use this column to find foods that are low in total fat. Generally, such foods include fruits, vegetables, grains, cereals, soy foods, fish, some poultry, and low-fat dairy. Highly refined or processed foods, meats, whole-milk dairy, baked goods, and snack foods typically have higher total fat (and usually high bad fat) content.

Good Fats

The "Good Fats" category includes the known values of monounsaturated and/or omega-3 fatty acids in the food or beverage. These are the healthy fats that benefit the heart, help lower cholesterol, and protect against insulin resistance. This value can help you choose foods that provide these advantages. Your intake of good fats should be 10 to 15 percent of your total daily calories. Based on the 2,000-calories-per-day model, your good fat intake should be 200 to 300 calories, as follows:

2,000 calories × 10% (or 15%) = 200 (or 300) ÷ 9 (number of calories in a gram of fat) = 22 (or 33) grams.

Bad Fats

This category contains the sum of saturated and trans fats in the food and beverages in the counter. These are the artery-clogging, heart-stopping fats, and the ones that you want to limit in your diet. Foods typically high in saturated fat include meats, butter, tropical oils, full-fat dairy products, margarine, and some processed foods. Trans fats are found in margarine, many processed foods such as snacks and crackers, packaged dinners, and fast foods.

Saturated and trans fat *together* should not exceed 10 percent of your total caloric intake per day. Given the standard 2,000 calories-per-day model, your daily intake of bad fats should not be more than 200 calories (2,000 calories × 10% = 200 ÷ 9 (number of calories in a gram of fat), or 22 grams. A quick look at the "Bad Fats" category will give you immediate information on the bad fat content of the foods and beverages you are considering and help you make healthier choices.

Fiber

This no-calorie nutrient plays many important roles in an anti-aging diet; for example, it helps re-duce cholesterol and triglyceride levels, fight obesity, prevent constipation, reduce risk of intestinal problems, including colon cancer, stabilize glucose levels, and remove toxins from the body. If you are between the ages of 19 and 50, you should strive to get 38 grams of fiber daily if you are male, and 25 grams if you are female. If you are older than 50, the National Academy of Sciences, Food and Nutrition Board recommends 30 grams for men and 21 grams for women.

You can scan the fiber column to find foods that contain a good fiber content (at least 2.5 to 3 grams per serving). Foods that typically fall into this range or higher include fruits and vegetables, cereals, grains, nuts, seeds, and some soy-based foods.

Sugar

Sugar refers to simple sugars, the ones that are especially harmful because they cause a rapid rise in blood glucose levels and lead to insulin resistance, both of which increase your risk of diabetes, heart disease, and many other serious medical conditions. High intake of simple sugars can also lead to weight gain.

Keep in mind that the "Sugars" category includes both naturally occurring sugars (like those found in fruit, fruit juices, milk, and some vegetables) as well as those that are added to foods and beverages. You can find added sugars on the ingredient lists on food packages.

You can use the "Sugars" category to help you limit the amount of added simple sugars in your diet and to ensure you get enough of the good sugars (complex carbs). When looking at foods that often have added sugars, such as breakfast cereals and cookies, you can scan the "Sugars" category for those that contain low amounts (between 0 and 5 grams of total sugars).

Beta-carotene

Beta-carotene is the most studied of the more than 600 different types of carotenoids that have been identified in plants. Carotenoids are pigments that give fruits and vegetables their color, and beta-carotene is an especially potent carotenoid. The role of beta-carotene in nature is to protect dark green, orange, and yellow fruits and vegetables from the damage caused by solar radiation, and it is believed it also helps protect the human body as well. The colors give you a clue as to the fruits and vegetables that contain high levels of this antioxidant, and they include yellow squash, cantaloupe, peaches, apricots, tomatoes, sweet potatoes, carrots, and green leafy vegetables.

Calcium

As you know, calcium is critical for strong bones, and an insufficient amount of calcium in the diet significantly increases the risk of osteoporosis and with it, an increased risk of fractures from falls. Therefore you should make every effort to make sure you are getting enough calcium in your diet (1,000 mg for men and women age 19 to 50 years;

1,200 mg for older adults). You can use the nutrition counter to help you identify the foods that are rich sources of this mineral. Some of those sources include dairy products, canned sardines, green leafy vegetables, yogurt, and soybeans.

Vitamin C

This potent antioxidant is an important member of the arsenal you should assemble in your fight against free radical damage and aging. Vitamin C (also known as ascorbic acid) is water soluble and is found in all body fluids. Because the body cannot store this antioxidant, it's very important to replenish your supply daily. When you use the nutrition counter, you will see that the best sources of vitamin C are fruits and fruit juices, vegetables and vegetable juices, and products that are enriched with vitamin C, including cereals.

In the nutrition counter, the vitamin C content per serving is given in DV. The Dietary Reference Intake (DRI, formerly RDA) is 75 mg for women and 90 mg for men; for smokers, 110 mg for women and 130 mg for men.

B vitamins

The B vitamins are essential to help preserve and maintain optimal function of the central nervous system and the production of neurotransmitters, which are critical for brain function because they carry signals from cell to cell. Generally, B vitamins help fight the signs and symptoms of an aging brain: for example, slowing of reflexes, difficulty recalling names or words, increasing bouts of forgetfulness and confusion, and episodes of mental "fog." B vitamins also play a critical role in the breakdown of carbohydrates into glucose (to provide energy), and in the maintenance of muscle tone in the gastrointestinal tract.

The vitamins that make up what is commonly called the "vitamin B complex" include thiamin (B1), riboflavin (B2), niacin (B3), pantothenic acid (B5), pyridoxine (B6), biotin (B7), folic acid (B9), and cobalamin (B12). Each of these vitamins has distinct characteristics, but they also have many similar properties and are found in many of the same common foods. At one time, this fact led researchers to consider them as one substance. For the sake of simplicity, we treat the B vitamins as a single entry for each food or beverage item and rate the vitamin B content as "0" for none or insignificant; "+" for a moderate amount, and "++" for a high amount.

Because the B vitamins are water soluble, they do not stay in the body very long (except for B12) and therefore need to be replenished regularly, preferably daily. You can use the information in this column to help you identify foods and beverages that contain these essential vitamins.

The information in the Anti-Aging Nutrition Counter was compiled from many sources, including but not limited to organizations within the United States government (Food and Drug Administration,

National Academy of Sciences, U.S. Department of Agriculture National Nutrient Database), individual food labels, food manufacturers, fast-food restaurants, and various Internet sources, including *Nutritiondata.com*. It's especially important to note that fast-food restaurants are constantly making adjustments to their menus, and so you may wish to ask about specific items to see if their nutritional content has changed.

This nutrition counter provides you with a wealth of information you need and can readily use to fight aging with every spoonful you take. Bring this book along with you to the supermarket, restaurants, farmers' markets—anywhere food is sold!

ABBREVIATIONS AND SYMBOLS

Here are the abbreviations and symbols you will see in the nutrition counter.

cont = container
g = gram
mcg = microgram
mg = milligram
mL = milliliters
Na = not available; the product may contain this substance but the manufacturer or company does not list this information on the label
oz = ounce
pc(s) = piece(s)
pkg = package

serv = serving

tbs = tablespoon

tsp = teaspoon

w = with

w/o = without

percentage DV = percent Daily Value, the recommended intake of a nutrient based on a 2,000 calorie diet

0 = none, zero, or an insignificant amount of B vitamins (<10% of two or more B vitamins)

+ = moderate amount of B vitamins (at least 10% of two or more B vitamins)

++ = high amount of B vitamins

* = the figure given is an estimate and based on similar, generic food items for which levels have been provided by the FDA. We provide this information because food manufacturers typically do not reveal beta carotene and B vitamin content on their labels. The specific brand-name food may contain the same or different amount of the nutrients.

Food	Portion Size	Calories	Total Fat (g)	Good Fats (g)	Bad Fats (g)	Fiber (g)	Sugars (mg)	Beta-carotene (mcg)	Calcium (%DV)	Vit. C (%DV)	B vit. (0,+,++)
ACORN SQUASH, boiled, mashed	½ c	42	0	0	0	3	0	2850	3	13	+
ALMONDS											
Dry roasted, no salt	1 oz	169	15	9.5	1	3	1	0.28	7	0	+
Oil roasted, no salt	1 oz	172	16	9.5	1	3	1	0.28	8	0	++
ANCHOVIES, in oil, drained	1 oz	59	3	1	1	0	0	0	6	0	0
APPLE JUICE											
Eden Foods, organic	8 oz	90	0	0	0	0	12	0	0	0	0
Minute Maid, frozen, prepared, fortified	8 oz	110	0	0	0	0	27	0	10	120	0
Minute Maid, apple white grape, box	200 mL	100	0	0	0	0	22	0	10	100	0
Mott's 100%, bottled	8 oz	120	0	0	0	0	28	0	2	20	0
Mott's Plus light juice beverage	8 oz	60	0	0	0	0	14	0	10	100	0
APPLESAUCE											
Eden Foods, organic	½ c	60	0	0	0	2	10	0	0	10	0
Mott's original	½ c	110	0	0	0	1	25	0	0	2	0
Mott's unsweetened	½ c	50	0	0	0	1	12	0	0	2	0
APPLES											
Raw, with skin	Medium	72	0	0	0	3	14	37	0	10	0
Raw, without skin	Medium	61	0	0	0	2	13	22	0	8	0
Dried, sulfured	1 c	209	0	0	0	7	49	0	1	5	0
APRICOTS, fresh	1	17	0	0	0	1	3	380	0	5	0
Dried	1 oz	68	0	0	0	9	69	2810	7	2	+
Del Monte, canned, halves, drained	½ c	100	0	0	0	1	25	2840	0	8	0
Del Monte, canned lite halves	½ c	60	0	0	0	1	15	2840	0	8	0

Food	Portion Size	Calories	Total Fat (g)	Good Fats (g)	Bad Fats (g)	Fiber (g)	Sugars (mg)	Beta-carotene (mcg)	Calcium (%DV)	Vit. C (%DV)	B vit. (0,+,++)
S&W, sun apricots	1/2 c	90	0	0	0	1	19	2840*	0	100	0
S&W whole	1/2 c	120	0	0	0	1	28	2840*	0	2	0
APRICOT NECTAR, organic (Santa Cruz)	8 oz	120	0	0	0	<1	27	1800	2	10	0
ARTICHOKE											
Globe or French, boiled	1	60	0	0	0	6	1	127	5	20	0
Birds Eye, hearts, frozen	12 pcs	40	1	0	0	5	0	Na	4	10	0
ASPARAGUS, fresh, cooked, no salt	1/2 c	20	0	0	0	2	1	543	2	11	+
Birds Eye, cuts, frozen	3/4 c	20	0	0	0	0	0	600*	0	15	+
Birds Eye, spears, frozen	7	20	0	0	0	0	0	290*	0	15	+
Del Monte, canned cuts & tips	1/2 c	20	0	0	0	1	0	1190*	0	25	+
Del Monte, canned, spears	7	20	0	0	0	1	0	540*	0	25	+
AVOCADO											
California	1	289	27	17	4	12	1	109	2	25	+
Florida	1	365	31	17	6	17	7	161	3	88	+‡
BACON											
Oscar Mayer, center cut	1/2 oz	50	4	Na	2	0	0	0	0	0	0
Oscar Mayer, hearty thick cut	3/4 oz	60	5	Na	1.5	0	0	0	0	0	0
Oscar Mayer, ready to serve	1/2 oz	70	5	Na	2	0	0	0	0	0	0
Oscar Mayer, ready to serve, Canadian	1 3/4 oz	60	2	Na	1	0	1	0	0	0	0
BACON SUBSTITUTE											
Morningstar Farms, strips	2 strips	60	4.5	1	0.5	<1	0	Na	0	0	+
Yves, Canadian veggie bacon	4 g	80	0.5	0	0	1	1	Na	2	0	+

87

Food	Portion Size	Calories	Total Fat (g)	Good Fats (g)	Bad Fats (g)	Fiber (g)	Sugars (mg)	Beta-carotene (mcg)	Calcium (%DV)	Vit. C (%DV)	B vit. (0,+,++)
BAGELS											
Pepperidge Farm, plain	1	260	1	0	0	5	9	Na	15	0	++
Pepperidge Farm, whole wheat	1	250	1.5	0	0	6	9	Na	15	0	++
Sara Lee											
Apple cinnamon, 4 oz	1	310	1.5	0	0	3	16	Na	15	0	+
Banana walnut, 4 oz	1	350	7	Na	2	4	10	Na	14	4	+
Blueberry, toaster size	1	160	0.5	0	0	1	4	Na	6	0	+
Cinnamon raisin, toaster size	1	160	0.5	0	0	1	3	Na	6	4	+
Cranberry orange, 4 oz	1	310	1.5	0	0	3	16	Na	14	4	+
Honey wheat, toaster size	1	250	1	0	0	4	7	Na	20	0	+
Onion, deluxe	1	260	1	0	0	2	5	Na	10	0	+
Plain, toaster size	1	160	0.5	0	0	1	3	Na	6	0	+
Sundried tomato & basil	1	300	1.5	0	0	2	6	Na	10	0	0
BANANA, raw, 7"	1	105	0	0	0	3	14	31	0	17	0
BARBEQUE SAUCE											
Hunts, original, bold	2 tbs	60	0	0	0	<1	11	0	0	0	0
Hunts, honey hickory	2 tbs	60	0	0	0	<1	11	0	0	0	0
Kraft, hickory smoke	2 tbs	40	0	0	0	0	7	0	0	0	0
Kraft, original	2 tbs	40	0	0	0	0	9	0	0	0	0
Kraft, thick spicy brown sugar	2 tbs	60	0	0	0	0	13	0	0	0	0
BARLEY, cooked	1 c	193	1	0	1	6	0	8	1	0	0
BASS, striped, cooked, dry heat	3 oz	105	3	1	1	0	0	0	1	0	‡

Food	Portion Size	Calories	Total Fat (g)	Good Fats (g)	Bad Fats (g)	Fiber (g)	Sugars (mg)	Beta-carotene (mcg)	Calcium (%DV)	Vit. C (%DV)	B vit. (0,+,++)
BEANS, baked											
B&M, maple flavor	½ c	160	1	0	0	8	12	0	6	0	+
Bush's Boston recipe	½ c	150	1	0	0	5	11	0	8	0	+
Campbell's pork 'n beans	½ c	140	1.5	1	0.5	7	0	0	6	4	+
S&W, country BBQ	½ c	140	0.5	0	0	6	11	0	6	0	+
S&W, honey mustard	½ c	140	0.5	0	0	6	11	0	8	0	+
S&W, sweet bacon	½ c	140	0.5	0	0	6	12	0	6	0	+
BEANS, other											
Adzuki, fresh, cooked w/salt	1 c	294	0	0	0	17	0	0	6	0	‡
Black, fresh, cooked w/salt	1 c	227	0	0	0	10	0	0	10	0	‡
Great northern, cooked, w/salt	1 c	209	1	0	0	12	0	0	12	3	‡
Navy, cooked w/salt	1 c	255	1	0	0	3	0	0	3	0	‡
Organic (Eden), adzuki	½ c	110	0	0	0	3	0	0	4	0	‡
Organic (Eden), black	½ c	110	1	0	0	6	0	0	6	0	‡
Organic (Eden), kidney	½ c	100	0	0	0	10	<1	0	6	0	‡
Organic (Eden), navy	½ c	110	1	0	0	6	<1	0	6	0	‡
Organic (Eden), pinto	½ c	110	1	0	0	6	<1	0	6	0	‡
Organic (Eden), soybeans, black	½ c	120	6	1.5	1	7	1	0	8	0	‡
S&W, black	½ c	70	0	0	0	6	1	0	6	4	‡
S&W, kidney	½ c	100	0.5	0	0	6	7	0	8	8	‡
S&W, white	½ c	80	0.5	0	0	6	1	0	6	0	+
BEEF											
Bottom sirloin, lean & fat, roasted, all grades	3 oz	177	9	4.5	3	0	0	0	0	0	‡
Bottom sirloin, lean, selected, roasted	3 oz	153	6	3	3	0	0	0	2	0	‡

Food	Portion Size	Calories	Total Fat (g)	Good Fats (g)	Bad Fats (g)	Fiber (g)	Sugars (mg)	Beta-carotene (mcg)	Calcium (%DV)	Vit. C (%DV)	B vit. (0,+,++)
Brisket, lean & fat, choice, braised, flat half	3 oz	186	9	4	3	0	0	0	1	0	‡‡
Brisket, lean, choice, braised	3 oz	180	7	3	3	0	0	0	1	0	‡‡
Chuck arm roast, lean & fat, choice, braised	3 oz	251	16	7	6	0	0	0	1	0	‡‡
Chuck blade roast, lean, choice, braised	3 oz	225	12	4	5	0	0	0	1	0	‡‡
Chuck blade roast, lean & fat, choice, braised	3 oz	296	22	9	9	0	0	0	1	0	‡‡
Corned beef brisket, cooked	3 oz	213	16	8	5	0	0	0	0	0	‡‡
Ground, 70% lean, pan-broiled	3 oz	202	13	6.5	5	0	0	0	3	0	‡‡
Ground, 85% lean, baked	3 oz	204	12	5.5	5	0	0	0	2	0	‡‡
Ground, 95% lean, baked	3 oz	148	5	2.5	2	0	0	0	0	0	‡‡
Liver, pan fried	3 oz	142	4	0.5	1	0	0	0	0	0	‡‡
Round, bottom, lean, choice, roasted	3 oz	157	6	2.5	2	0	0	0	0	0	‡‡
Short loin, lean & fat, choice, broiled	3 oz	241	17	8	6	0	0	0	0	0	‡‡
Short loin, lean, choice, broiled	3 oz	190	11	5	4	0	0	0	0	0	‡‡
Top sirloin, lean & fat, choice, broiled	3 oz	186	9	4	3	0	0	0	1	0	‡‡
Top sirloin, lean, choice, broiled	3 oz	160	6	2	2	0	0	0	1	0	‡‡
BEEF SUBSTITUTES											
Amy's Kitchen, All American burger	1	120	3	Na	0	3	2	0	4	6	Na
Amy's Kitchen, California veg burger	1	140	5	Na	0.5	4	2	0	4	6	Na
Amy's Kitchen, Chicago veg burger	1	160	5	Na	1.5	3	2	0	8	4	Na
Amy's Kitchen, Texas veg burger	1	120	2.5	Na	0	3	2	0	4	2	Na
Boca Burgers, organic cheeseburger	1	120	4.5	Na	2	3	1	0	8	0	+
Boca Burgers, organic vegan	1	100	2.5	Na	0	4	0	0	6	0	+

Food	Portion Size	Calories	Total Fat (g)	Good Fats (g)	Bad Fats (g)	Fiber (g)	Sugars (mg)	Beta-carotene (mcg)	Calcium (%DV)	Vit. C (%DV)	B vit. (0,+,++)
Boca Burgers, roasted garlic	1	70	1.5	Na	0	4	0	0	6	0	+
Boca Burgers, onion	1	70	1	Na	0	4	1	0	10	0	+
Morningstar Grillers, vegan	1 patty	100	2.5	1	0.5	4	0	0	4	0	‡‡
Morningstar Burger Crumbles	1 cup	165	5	1	0.5	4.5	1	0	6	0	+
Morningstar Garden veggie burger	1 patty	100	2.5	0.5	0.5	4	0	265	4	0	‡‡
Morningstar Grillers, original	1 patty	130	6	2	1	2	<1	0	4	0	Na
Morningstar Mushroom lover's burger	1 patty	110	6	2	1	<1	1	0	4	0	+
Morningstar Spicy black bean burger	1 patty	140	4.5	1	0.5	5	2	0	8	0	+
Morningstar Steak strips	12 strips	150	3.5	1.5	0.5	3	1	0	4	0	+
Worthington dinner roast	3/4" slice	180	11	4.5	1.5	3	1	0	2	0	+
Worthington meatless corned beef	3 slices	140	9	2	1	0	1	0	2	0	‡‡
Worthington Redi-Burger patties 5/8"	1 patty	120	2.5	0.5	0.5	4	1	0	0	0	+
Worthington Swiss steak	1 pc	130	6	1.5	1	3	<1	0	0	0	+
Worthington Tender Rounds	6 pcs	120	4.5	1.5	0.5	1	1	0	2	0	+
Worthington Vege-Burger	1/4 c	60	0.5	0	0	2	0	0	0	0	+
Worthington vegetarian burger	1/4 c	70	1.5	0	0	1	0	0	0	0	+
BEER											
Beer, light	12 oz	103	0	0	0	0	0	0	0	0	0
Beer, nonalcoholic	12 oz	70	0	0	0	0	0	0	0	0	0
Beer, regular	12 oz	153	0	0	0	0	0	0	0	0	0
BEETS, fresh, boiled, sliced	1/2 c	37	0	0	0	2	7	18	1	5	0
Del Monte, canned, sliced	1/2 c	35	0	0	0	2	5	25	0	4	0
Del Monte, pickled	1/2 c	80	0	0	0	2	16	0	0	6	0

Food	Portion Size	Calories	Total Fat (g)	Good Fats (g)	Bad Fats (g)	Fiber (g)	Sugars (mg)	Beta-carotene (mcg)	Calcium (%DV)	Vit. C (%DV)	B vit. (0, +, ++)
BISCUITS											
Bisquick (box/mix)											
Complete buttermilk, mix	1/3 c	150	7	Na	5	<1	1	0	4	0	+
Complete cheese garlic, mix	1/3 c	160	7	Na	5	<1	2	0	4	0	0
Heart smart, mix	1/3 c	140	2.5	1.5	0	1	3	0	20	0	+
Honey butter, mix	1/3 c	160	6	Na	4.5	0	6	0	2	0	0
Original, mix	1/3 c	160	5	Na	3	1	1	0	4	0	+
Pillsbury (refrigerated)											
Freezer to Oven, buttermilk	1	200	10	Na	6.5	<1	2	0	2	0	0
Freezer to Oven, cheddar garlic	1	190	9	Na	6	<1	3	0	2	0	0
Freezer to Oven, southern	1	180	9	Na	6.5	<1	2	0	2	0	0
Grands buttermilk	1	190	8.5	Na	6	1	4	0	2	0	0
Grands, extra rich	1	210	10	Na	7.5	<1	6	0	4	0	0
Grands, flaky layers, buttermilk	1	190	9	Na	5.5	<1	5	0	2	0	0
BLACKBERRIES, fresh	1 c	62	1	0	0	8	7	184	4	50	0
BLUEBERRIES, fresh	1 c	83	0	0	0	2	14	46	0	23	0
Cascadian Farm, frozen	1 c	70	1	0	0	4	12	43*	0	4	0
Dole, frozen	1 c	70	0	0	0	4	12	43*	0	6	0
BLUEFISH, baked	3 oz	135	5	2	1	0	0	0	0	0	‡
BOK CHOY, cooked, shredded	1 c	20	0	0	0	2	1	4333	15	73	+
BOLOGNA											
Louis Rich, turkey bologna	1 slice	50	4	Na	1	0	0	0	4	0	0
Oscar Mayer, beef	1 slice	90	8	Na	4	0	1	0	0	0	0

Food	Portion Size	Calories	Total Fat (g)	Good Fats (g)	Bad Fats (g)	Fiber (g)	Sugars (mg)	Beta-carotene (mcg)	Calcium (%DV)	Vit. C (%DV)	B vit. (0,+,++)
Oscar Mayer, beef light	1 slice	56	4	Na	2	0	1	0	0	0	0
Oscar Mayer, fat free	1 slice	20	0	0	0	0	1	0	2	0	0
BOUILLON/BROTH											
College Inn											
Beef	1 c	25	1	0	0	0	0	0	2	0	0
Beef, French onion style	1 c	15	0	0	0	0	0	0	0	0	0
Chicken	1 c	15	0	0	0	0	0	0	0	0	0
Chicken w/lemon & herb	1 c	15	1	0	0	0	0	0	0	0	0
Turkey	1 c	20	1	0	0	0	0	0	0	0	0
Imagine											
Organic beef	1 c	20	1	0	0	0	1	0	0	2	0
Organic free-range chicken	1 c	10	0	0	0	0	0	0	4	0	0
Organic low-sodium vegetable	1 c	20	0	0	0	<1	1	0	2	0	0
Organic no chicken	1 c	10	0	0	4	0	1	0	2	0	0
BRAZIL NUTS, unblanched, dried	1 oz	185	19	7	4	2	1	0	4	0	0
BREADS											
Earth Grains											
Buttermilk	1 slice	110	1.5	0	0	<1	4	Na	10	0	+
Honey wheat berry	1 slice	100	0.5	0	0	1	2	Na	10	0	+
Honey whole grain	1 slice	120	1.5	0	0	2	3	Na	10	0	0
Oat & nut	1 slice	120	2.5	0	0.5	1	4	Na	10	0	+
Potato	1 slice	110	1	0	0	<1	3	Na	10	0	+
100% multigrain	1 slice	110	1.5	0	0	5	3	Na	15	0	+
100% whole wheat stone ground	1 slice	100	1	0	0	2	3	Na	10	0	0

Food	Portion Size	Calories	Total Fat (g)	Good Fats (g)	Bad Fats (g)	Fiber (g)	Sugars (mg)	Beta-carotene (mcg)	Calcium (%DV)	Vit. C (%DV)	B vit. (0,+,++)
Oroweat											
Buttermilk, country	1 slice	100	1	0	0	<1	4	0	2	0	0
Honey fiber whole grain	1 slice	80	1	0	0	4	3	0	15	0	+
Oatnut	1 slice	100	1.5	Na	0.5	1	3	0	0	0	0
Whole grain nut	1 slice	90	1.5	Na	0	3	3	0	4	0	0
Whole wheat	1 slice	100	1	Na	0	3	4	0	6	0	0
Pepperidge Farm											
9 Grain natural whole grain	1 slice	100	2	Na	0	3	3	0	4	0	0
German dark wheat	1 slice	100	1.5	Na	0	3	3		4		0
Honey whole wheat	1 slice	110	2	Na	0.5	3	4	0	4	0	0
Multigrain, whole grain	1 slice	120	2	Na	0	3	3	0	4	0	0
Oatmeal whole grain	1 slice	110	2	Na	0.5	3	3	0	4	0	0
Soft honey wheat	2 slices	160	2	Na	0.5	4	4	0	10	2	0
Whole grain cinnamon swirl	1 slice	100	1.5	Na	0	2	5	0	2	2	+
Whole grain white Farmhouse	1 slice	110	2	Na	0.5	3	4	0	10	0	0
Sara Lee											
100% whole wheat	1 slice	70	1	0.5	0	2	3	0	10	0	+
Delightful white	2 slices	90	1	0	0	4	1	0	6	0	0
Heart healthy multigrain	1 slice	100	0.5	0	0	2	4	0	6	0	0
Honey wheat	1 slice	90	1	0	0	1	2	0	6	0	0
BREAD CRUMBS											
Garlic & herb (Progresso)	¼ c	110	1.5	0	1.5	1	2	0	4	0	0
Italian style (Progresso)	¼ c	110	1.5	0	1.5	1	2	0	4	0	0
Plain (Progresso)	¼ c	110	1.5	0	1.5	1	2	0	4	0	0

Food	Portion Size	Calories	Total Fat (g)	Good Fats (g)	Bad Fats (g)	Fiber (g)	Sugars (mg)	Beta-carotene (mcg)	Calcium (%DV)	Vit. C (%DV)	B vit. (0,+,++)
BROCCOLI, fresh, boiled, chopped	½ c	27	0	0	0	3	1	920	3	54	0
Frozen, Birds Eye											
Florets	1 c	30	0	0	0	2	0	900*	2	50	0
With cheese sauce	½ c	90	5	Na	3	1	0	450*	6	40	0
With beans, peppers, onions	1 c	30	0	0	0	2	0	Na	2	25	0
With corn & peppers	¾ c	60	1	0	0	1	0	Na	2	30	0
With peppers, onion, mushrooms	1 c	30	0	0	0	1	0	Na	2	45	0
With cauliflower & peppers	1 c	25	0	0	0	1	0	Na	2	45	0
Frozen, Green Giant											
Spears in butter	4 oz	40	1.5	0.5	1	2	3	600*	2	60	0
With cauliflower, carrots, cheese	⅔ c	60	2.5	0.5	1	2	3	Na	4	30	0
With cheese	⅔ c	60	2.5	0.5	1	2	2	Na	6	45	0
With zesty cheese	¾ c	60	2	Na	0.5	1	4	Na	4	35	Na
BRUSSELS SPROUTS, fresh, boiled	½ c	28	0	0	0	2	1	0	2	80	0
Frozen (Birds Eye)	10 pcs	45	0	0	0	3	0	0	2	90	0
Frozen, w/cauliflower & carrots (Birds Eye)	1 c	40	0	0	0	2	0	0	2	60	0
With butter sauce (Green Giant)	½ c	60	1	0	0.5	3	3	-1	2	90	0
BULGUR, cooked	1 c	151	0	0	0	8	0	0	1	0	0
BUTTER, regular salted	1 tbs	100	11	3	7	0	0	22	0	0	0
Whipped, salted	1 tbs	66	8	2	5	0	0	14	0	0	0
BUTTERMILK, lowfat	8 oz	98	2	0	1	0	12	2	28	4	0
CABBAGE											
Green, raw, shredded	½ c	8	0	0	0	1	0	0	1	29	0
Green, boiled, no salt, shredded	½ c	16	0	0	0	1	2	55	2	25	0

Food	Portion Size	Calories	Total Fat (g)	Good Fats (g)	Bad Fats (g)	Fiber (g)	Sugars (mg)	Beta-carotene (mcg)	Calcium (%DV)	Vit. C (%DV)	B vit. (0,+,++)
Napa, cooked	1 c	13	0	0	0	0	0	145	2	5	0
Red, raw, chopped	1 c	28	0	0	0	2	3	596	4	84	0
Red, boiled, shredded	1 c	44	0	0	0	4	2	0	4	84	0
Savoy, raw, shredded	1 c	19	0	0	0	2	2	420	2	36	0
Savoy, boiled, shredded	1 c	35	0	0	0	4	0	0	4	41	+
CAKE, boxed mix (mix only) Betty Crocker											
Angel food confetti	1/12 mix	150	0	0	0	0	24	0	6	0	0
Angel food white	1/12 mix	140	0	0	0	0	23	0	6	0	0
Brownie, fudge, chewy	1/20 mix	100	1	0	0	1	15	0	0	0	0
Brownie, fudge, low fat, prep.	1/18	130	2.5	1	1.5	1	18	0	2	0	0
Brownie, supreme, frosted	1/20 mix	150	3	Na	2	1	22	0	2	0	0
Brownie, supreme, turtle	1/20 mix	120	2.5	Na	0.5	<1	16	0	0	0	0
Complete Desserts, hot fudge cake	1/6 mix	440	13	Na	7	3	53	0	40	0	0
Gingerbread cake & cookie mix	1/8 mix	210	5	1.5	3	0	19	0	6	0	0
Pineapple upside down cake	1/6 mix	350	9	3	5.5	0	43	0	4	0	0
Pound cake	1/8 mix	240	7	1.5	4	0	26	0	4	0	0
Quick bread, banana	1/12 mix	130	2.5	Na	1.5	0	13	0	0	0	0
Quick bread, cinnamon streusel	1/14 mix	160	4	Na	2	0	15	0	2	0	0
Quick bread, cranberry orange	1/12 mix	150	3	Na	1.5	<1	16	0	0	0	0
Super Moist											
Butter pecan	1/12 mix	170	3	1	2.5	0	19	0	6	0	0
Butter recipe, white	1/12	170	3	1	1.5	0	20	0	4	0	0
Carrot	1/12 mix	200	3	Na	2	0	2	0	10	0	0
Chocolate fudge	1/12 mix	170	3	Na	2	1	18	0	4	0	0

96

Food	Portion Size	Calories	Total Fat (g)	Good Fats (g)	Bad Fats (g)	Fiber (g)	Sugars (mg)	Beta-carotene (mcg)	Calcium (%DV)	Vit. C (%DV)	B vit. (0,+,++)
Cinnamon swirl	1/12 mix	200	3.5	1	2	0	25	0	8	0	0
French vanilla	1/12 mix	170	3.5	1	2	0	18	0	6	0	0
German chocolate	1/12 mix	170	3	Na	2	1	18	0	4	0	0
Lemon	1/12 mix	170	3.5	1	2	0	18	0	4	0	0
Party rainbow chip	1/10 mix	210	4	Na	2.5	1	18	0	4	0	0
Yellow	1/12 mix	170	3.5	Na	2	0	18	0	6	0	0

CAKE, Snack

Tastykake

Food	Portion Size	Calories	Total Fat (g)	Good Fats (g)	Bad Fats (g)	Fiber (g)	Sugars (mg)	Beta-carotene (mcg)	Calcium (%DV)	Vit. C (%DV)	B vit. (0,+,++)
Banana Kreamies, family pack	1 pc	170	8	Na	4	0	18	Na	2	0	0
Butterscotch Filled Krimpets, family pack	2 pcs	210	6	Na	3	0	26	Na	2	0	0
Chocolate cupcakes, family pack	2 pcs	210	7	Na	3	2	26	Na	2	0	0
Chocolate Kandy Kakes, family pack	2 pcs	180	10	Na	7	1	17	Na	2	0	0
Chocolate Kreme filled Krimpets, family pack	2 pcs	190	4	Na	1.5	0	25	Na	2	0	0
Chocolate Kreamies, family pack	1 pc	190	9	Na	4.5	0	18	Na	4	0	0
Chocolate Junior, single serve	2 pc	340	12	Na	6	1	37	Na	2	0	0
Cream filled chocolate cupcakes, family pack	2 pcs	250	10	Na	4.5	0	27	Na	2	0	0
Cream filled Koffee cake cupcakes	2 pcs	270	13	Na	2.5	0	22	Na	2	0	0
Glazed Honey Bun, family pack	1 pc	330	18	Na	11	<1	19	Na	8	4	0
Koffee Kake Jr, single serve	1 pc	280	10	Na	3.5	<1	25	Na	4	0	0
Peanut butter Kandy Kake, family pack	2 pcs	180	10	Na	5	1	14	Na	2	0	0

CANDY

Food	Portion Size	Calories	Total Fat (g)	Good Fats (g)	Bad Fats (g)	Fiber (g)	Sugars (mg)	Beta-carotene (mcg)	Calcium (%DV)	Vit. C (%DV)	B vit. (0,+,++)
Almond Joy (Hershey)	45 g	220	12	Na	8	2	24	0	3	0	0
Caramello	6 blocks	200	9	2	6	1	24	0	9	1	0
Chocolate bar, milk w/almonds	41 g	230	14	5	6	1	17	0	8	1	0

Food	Portion Size	Calories	Total Fat (g)	Good Fats (g)	Bad Fats (g)	Fiber (g)	Sugars (mg)	Beta-carotene (mcg)	Calcium (%DV)	Vit. C (%DV)	B vit. (0,+,++)
5th Avenue	2 oz	280	14	5	5	2	26	0	4	0	0
Goobers	10 pcs	51	3	1.5	1	1	0	0	1	0	0
Heath Toffee bar	39 g	220	13	3	7	1	23	0	3	0	0
Kit Kat, 4-piece bar	1	220	11	2.5	7	0	20	0	5	0	0
Krackel	41 g	210	10	2.5	6	1	22	0	6	0	0
M&Ms	1.69 oz	240	10	1.5	6	1	31	0	5	0	0
M&M peanut	1.74 oz	250	13	5	5	2	25	0	4	0	0
Mr. Goodbar	49 g	270	16	4	7	2	23	0	5	0	0
Raisinets	10 pcs	41	2	0.5	1	1	0	0	1	0	0
Reese's Nut Rageous	51 g	280	16	7	5	2	22	0	3	0	0
Reese's Pieces	43 g	220	11	2	7	1	29	0	3	0	0
Rolo	48 g	210	9	1.5	7	0	27	0	6	0	0
Skor	39 g	210	12	3.5	7	1	23	0	6	0	0
Symphony, milk chocolate	42 g	230	13	3.5	8	1	23	0	10	1	0
Tootsie Roll	6 pcs	155	1	1	0	0	23	0	1	0	0
Twizzlers, strawberry	2.5 oz	249	2	0	0	0	23	0	0	0	0
York peppermint patty	39 g	160	3	0	1.5	1	27	0	0	0	0
CANTALOUPE, raw, cubed	1 c	54	0	0	0	1	13	3232	1	97	0
CARROTS											
Raw, large 7–8.5"	1	30	0	0	0	2	3	4157	2	7	0
Cooked, no salt, slices	½ c	27	0	0	0	2	3	6410	2	4	0
Birds Eye, frozen, sliced	⅔ c	35	0	0	0	2	0	7800*	2	2	0
Del Monte, canned	½ c	35	0	0	0	3	5	7700*	2	6	0
Del Monte, canned, honey glazed	½ c	70	0	0	0	1	12	7700*	4	10	0

Food	Portion Size	Calories	Total Fat (g)	Good Fats (g)	Bad Fats (g)	Fiber (g)	Sugars (mg)	Beta-carotene (mcg)	Calcium (%DV)	Vit. C (%DV)	B vit. (0,+,++)
CARROT JUICE											
Odwalla	8 oz	70	0	0	0	1	13	21,900*	4	0	0
Hain w/lutein	8 oz	80	0.5	0	0	0	11	21,900*	15	20	0
CASABA MELON, raw cubes	1 c	48	0	0	0	2	10	0	1	61	0
CASHEWS, dry roast, no salt	1 oz	162	13	7.5	3	1	1	0	1	0	0
CASHEW BUTTER, Maranatha	2 tbs	190	15	9	3	2	2	0	8	0	+
CAULIFLOWER, raw	1 c	25	0	0	0	3	2	8	2	77	0
Boiled, no salt	1 c	28	0	0	0	4	2	4	2	45	0
Birds Eye, frozen, florets	4 pcs	25	0	0	0	1	0	4*	0	35	0
Birds Eye, cauliflower, carrots & snow peas	1 c	30	0	0	0	2	0	Na	2	20	0
Green Giant, cauliflower & cheese sauce	½ c	50	2.5	0.5	1	1	2	Na	4	25	0
CELERY, raw, 7–8" stalk	1 stalk	6	0	0	0	1	1	108	1	2	0
CEREAL, cold/dry, ready-to-eat											
Arrowhead Mills											
Amaranth flakes	1 c	140	2	0.5	0	3	4	0	2	30	0
Kamut flakes	1 c	120	1	0	0.5	2	2	0	2	20	0
Multigrain flakes	1 c	170	2	0.5	0	3	3	0	2	25	0
Organic nature Os	1 c	130	2	0.5	0.5	2	1	0	0	10	0
Puffed corn	1 c	50	0	Na	0	2	0	0	0	0	0
Puffed millet	1 c	50	0.5	0.5	0	1	0	0	0	0	0
Rice flakes, sweetened	1 c	180	1	0.5	0	1	8	0	0	35	0
Sweetened shredded wheat	1 c	200	1	0	0	5	12	0	2	0	0

Food	Portion Size	Calories	Total Fat (g)	Good Fats (g)	Bad Fats (g)	Fiber (g)	Sugars (mg)	Beta-carotene (mcg)	Calcium (%DV)	Vit. C (%DV)	B vit. (0,+,++)
Barbara's Bakery											
Alpen, original	2/3 c	200	3	0	0	4	11	Na	6	25	++
Brown rice crisps	1 c	120	1	0	0	1	2	Na	0	0	0
Honey Nut O's, organic	3/4 c	2	Na	0	8	2	11	Na	8	25	++
Organic Wild Puffs, caramel	3/4 c	110	1	Na	0	<1	9	Na	4	25	++
Puffins, original	3/4 c	90	1	Na	0	5	5	Na	0	10	Na
Shredded oats	1 1/4 c	220	2.5	Na	0.5	5	12	Na	2	35	+
General Mills											
Apple cinnamon Cheerios	3/4 c	120	1.5	1	0	1	13	Na	10	100	+
Cheerios	1 c	100	2	0.5	0	1	1	Na	10	10	+
Cheerios, honey nut	3/4 c	110	1.5	0.5	0	2	9	Na	10	10	+
Cheerios, multigrain	1 c	110	1	0	0	3	6	Na	10	25	++
Basic 4	1 c	200	3	1	1.5	3	14	Na	25	0	+
Cinnamon Toast Crunch	3/4 c	130	3	2	0.5	1	10	Na	10	0	+
Cocoa Puffs	1 c	110	1.5	0.5	1	1	12	Na	10	0	+
Corn Chex	1 c	120	0.5	0	0	1	3	Na	10	10	+
Country corn flakes	1 c	120	0.5	0	0	1	3	Na	25	10	+
Fiber One	1/2 c	60	1	0	0	14	0	Na	10	10	+
Golden Grahams	3/4 c	120	1	0.5	0	1	11	Na	10	10	+
Kix	1 1/4 c	110	1	0	0	3	3	Na	15	10	+
Lucky Charms	3/4 c	110	1	0	0	1	12	Na	10	10	+
Oatmeal Crisp w/almonds	1 c	240	5	2.5	0.5	4	16	Na	4	0	+
Raisin nut bran	1 c	180	3	1.5	0.5	4	16	Na	2	0	+
Rice Chex	1 1/4 c	120	0.5	0	0	0	2	Na	10	10	+

Food	Portion Size	Calories	Total Fat (g)	Good Fats (g)	Bad Fats (g)	Fiber (g)	Sugars (mg)	Beta-carotene (mcg)	Calcium (%DV)	Vit. C (%DV)	B vit. (0,+,++)
Total, whole grain	¾ c	100	1.5	0	0	3	5	Na	100	100	‡
Trix	1 c	120	1.5	0	0	1	13	Na	10	10	+
Wheaties	¾ c	100	0.5	0	0	3	4	Na	2	10	‡
Kashi											
GoLean	1 c	140	1	Na	0	6	10	6	0	0	0
Good Friends	1 c	170	2	Na	0	2	12	9	0	0	0
Heart to Heart, honey	¾ c	110	1.5	Na	0	0	5	5	50	Na	‡
Organic Promise, Autumn Wheat	1 c	190	1	Na	0	3	6	7	3	0	0
Organic Promise, Cranberry	1 c	92	1	0	0	0	7	0	0	0	0
Organic Promise, Strawberry Fields	1 c	111	0	0	0	1	9	0	0	0	0
Seven in the Morning	1 c	207	2	0.5	0	7	3	0	2	0	0
Kelloggs											
All-Bran Buds	⅓ c	70	1	0	0	3	8	0	1	0	‡
Apple Jacks	1 c	130	0.5	0	0	1	6	0	0	25	+
Cocoa Krispies	¾ c	120	1	0	0.5	1	14	0	4	25	+
Complete Oat Bran Flakes	¾ c	110	1	0	0	4	6	0	0	100	‡
Corn Flakes	1 c	100	0	0	0	1	2	0	0	10	+
Corn Pops	1 c	117	0	0	0	<1	14	0	0	10	+
Cracklin' Oat Bran	¾ c	220	7	4.5	3	6	15	0	2	25	+
Froot Loops	1 c	120	1	0	0.5	1	15	0	0	25	+
Frosted Flakes	¾ c	120	0	0	0	1	12	0	0	10	+
Frosted Mini Wheats, bite-size	24 pcs	200	1	0	0	6	12	0	0	0	‡
Low-Fat Granola w/raisins	⅔ c	230	3	1.5	1	3	18	0	2	2	‡
Mueslix	⅔ c	200	3	1.5	0	4	17	0	3	0	‡

Food	Portion Size	Calories	Total Fat (g)	Good Fats (g)	Bad Fats (g)	Fiber (g)	Sugars (mg)	Beta-carotene (mcg)	Calcium (%DV)	Vit. C (%DV)	B vit. (0,+,++)
Product 19	1 c	100	0	0	0	1	4	20	0	100	‡
Raisin Bran	1 c	190	1.5	0.5	0	7	20	0	2	0	0
Rice Krispies	1¼ c	120	0	0	0	0	4	0	0	0	+
Rice Krispies Treat Cereal	¾ c	120	1.5	0.5	0	0	9	0	0	10	+
Smart Start Antioxidants	1 c	190	0.5	0	0	3	14	0	1	25	‡
Special K	1 c	110	0	0	0	1	4	0	0	34	‡
Malt-O-Meal											
Coco Roos	¾ c	120	1.5	0	0	<1	15	0	10	10	+
Colossal Crunch	¾ c	120	1.5	0	0	0	13	0	0	0	+
Crispy Rice	1¼ c	130	0	0	0	0	3	0	0	25	+
Frosted Flakes	¾ c	120	0	0	0	1	12	0	0	25	‡
Frosted Mini Spooners	1 c	190	1	0	0	6	11	0	0	0	‡
Marshmallow Mateys	1 c	120	1	0	0	1	13	0	10	10	+
Raisin Bran	1 c	220	1	0	0	7	21	0	2	0	+
Tootie Fruities	1 c	130	1	0	0	1	15	0	10	25	+
Post											
Alpha Bits, no sugar	1 oz	110	2	Na	0	3	0	0	10	10	Na
Banana Nut Crunch	2 oz	240	6	Na	1	4	12	0	2	0	+
Bran Flakes	1 oz	100	0.5	Na	0	5	5	0	0	0	+
Cocoa Pebbles	1 oz	110	1.5	Na	1	3	9	0	2	0	+
Fruit & Bran	2 oz	200	3	Na	0	6	15	0	0	0	+
Golden Crisp	1 oz	110	0	Na	0	1	14	0	0	0	+
Grape Nuts	2 oz	200	1	Na	0	6	5	0	2	0	+
Grape Nuts Flakes	1 oz	110	1	Na	0	3	4	0	0	0	+

Food	Portion Size	Calories	Total Fat (g)	Good Fats (g)	Bad Fats (g)	Fiber (g)	Sugars (mg)	Beta-carotene (mcg)	Calcium (%DV)	Vit. C (%DV)	B vit. (0,+,++)
Honey Bunches of Oats, honey roasted	1 oz	120	1.5	Na	0	2	6	0	0	0	+
Honey Bunches of Oats, Strawberry	1 oz	120	2	Na	0	2	8	0	0	6	+
Honey Comb	1 oz	120	1	Na	0	3	10	0	0	0	+
Quaker											
Life, cinnamon	¾ c	120	1.5	0.5	0	2	8	0	10	0	‡
Life, honey graham	¾ c	120	1.5	0.5	0	2	7	0	10	0	‡
Life, original	¾ c	120	1.5	0.5	0	2	6	6	11	0	‡
Mothers Toasted Oat Bran	¾ c	120	1.5	0.5	0	3	5	0	2	0	0
CEREALS, hot											
Arrowhead Mills											
4 Grains plus Flax	¼ c	140	1.5	0.5	0	9	0	0	2	0	0
Bear Mush	¼ c	150	1	0	0	2	0	0	15	0	0
Oat Flakes	⅓ c	130	2	0.5	0.5	4	0	0	2	0	+
Rice and Shine	¼ c	150	1	0.5	0	2	<1	0	0	0	+
Yellow corn grits	¼ c	130	0	0	0	1	0	0	0	0	0
Cream of Wheat											
Apple & cinnamon instant	1 pkt	130	0	0	0	1	16	0	20	0	+
Cinnamon swirl	1 pkt	130	0	0	0	1	14	0	20	0	+
Maple brown sugar	1 pkt	120	0	0	0	1	13	0	20	0	+
Quaker											
Instant, apples & cinnamon	1 pkt	130	1.5	0.5	0.5	3	12	0	10	0	+
Instant, maple & brown sugar	1 pkt	160	2	1	0	3	13	0	10	0	+
Nutrition for Women, golden brown sugar	1 pkt	170	2	1	0.5	3	12	0	50	0	+
Nutrition for Women, vanilla cinnamon	1 pkt	160	2	0.5	0.5	3	13	0	50	0	+

Food	Portion Size	Calories	Total Fat (g)	Good Fats (g)	Bad Fats (g)	Fiber (g)	Sugars (mg)	Beta-carotene (mcg)	Calcium (%DV)	Vit. C (%DV)	B vit. (0,+,++)
Oatmeal, Express baked apple	1 c	200	2.5	Na	0.5	4	19	0	10	10	+
Oatmeal, Express cinnamon roll	1 c	210	3.5	Na	0.5	4	17	0	10	0	+
Quick Oats, dry	½ c	150	3	1	0.5	4	1	0	0	0	0
CEREAL BARS											
Barbara's Bakery											
Fruit & yogurt bars, apple cinnamon	1	150	3	Na	0	1	15	0	25	10	+
Fruit & yogurt bars, blueberry apple	1	150	3	Na	0	1	15	0	25	10	+
Fruit & yogurt bars, cherry apple	1	150	3	Na	0	1	15	0	25	10	+
Granola, oats & honey	1	80	2	Na	0	<1	6	0	2	<2	0
Granola, peanut butter	1	80	3	Na	0	<1	14	0	0	0	Na
Puffins, Cereal & milk, blueberry	1	130	1.5	Na	1	3	8	0	30	30	+
Puffins, Cereal & milk, French toast	1	130	1.5	Na	1	3	7	0	30	30	+
Puffins, Cereal & milk, peanut butter, choc	1	140	3.5	Na	2	3	7	0	30	30	+
Cascadian Farm											
Granola, chocolate chip	1	140	3	Na	1	1	10	0	0	0	0
Granola, fruit & nut	1	140	4	Na	1	1	11	0	0	0	0
Granola, harvest berries	1	130	2	Na	0	1	13	0	0	0	0
Granola, multigrain	1	130	2	Na	0	1	9	0	0	0	0
Kelloggs											
Nutri-Grain, apple cinnamon	1	140	3	Na	0.5	1	13	0	20	0	+
Nutri-Grain, cherry	1	140	3	Na	0.5	<1	14	0	20	0	+
Nutri-Grain, fruit & nut, cranberry, raisin	1	120	3.5	Na	1	3	11	0	0	0	+

Food	Portion Size	Calories	Total Fat (g)	Good Fats (g)	Bad Fats (g)	Fiber (g)	Sugars (mg)	Beta-carotene (mcg)	Calcium (%DV)	Vit. C (%DV)	B vit. (0,+,++)
Nature Valley											
Apple Crisp	2 bars	180	6	Na	0.5	2	11	0	0	0	+
Maple brown sugar	2 bars	180	6	Na	0.5	2	11	0	0	0	+
Oats & honey	2 bars	180	6	Na	0.5	2	11	0	0	0	+
CHEESE											
American, 2% milk, singles (Kraft)	1 slice	45	3	Na	1.5	0	1	14*	20	0	0
American, singles (Kraft)	1 slice	60	4.5	Na	2.5	0	1	17*	20	0	0
American, Deli Deluxe (Kraft)	1 slice	80	7	2	4	0	0	17*	25	0	0
American (Land-O-Lakes)	1 oz	110	9	NA	6	0	1	17*	15	0	0
American, burger deli style (Sargento)	1 slice	70	6	Na	3.5	0	0	17*	15	0	0
Camembert	1 oz	85	7	2	4	0	0	3	10	0	0
Cheddar, mild (Organic Valley)	1 oz	110	9	2.5	6	0	0	23*	20	0	0
Cheddar, sharp (Organic Valley)	1 oz	110	9	2.5	6	0	0	23*	20	0	0
Cheddar, sharp deli style sliced (Sargento)	1 slice	80	6	2.5	4	0	0	23*	15	0	0
Colby (Organic Valley)	1 oz	110	9	Na	6	0	<1	12*	20	0	0
Colby, deli style sliced (Sargento)	1 slice	80	7	Na	4	0	0	12*	15	0	0
Cottage Cheese											
Breakstone, small curd, fat free	5 oz	80	0	0	0	0	6	5*	15	0	0
Breakstone, large curd, 2%	4 oz	90	2.5	0.5	1.5	0	5	5*	15	0	0
Breakstone, small curd, 4%	4 oz	120	5	Na	1.5	0	5	5*	15	0	0
Breakstone, Cottage Doubles, apples & cinn.	5.5 oz	140	2.5	Na	1.5	0	5	Na	8	0	0
Breakstone, Cottage Doubles, blueberry	5.5 oz	140	2.5	Na	1.5	0	14	Na	5	0	0
Breakstone, Cottage Doubles, peach	5.5 oz	130	2	Na	1.5	0	14	Na	15	0	0
Breakstone, Cottage Doubles, strawberry	5.5 oz	130	2	Na	1.5	0	15	Na	5	6	0

105

Food	Portion Size	Calories	Total Fat (g)	Good Fats (g)	Bad Fats (g)	Fiber (g)	Sugars (mg)	Beta-carotene (mcg)	Calcium (%DV)	Vit. C (%DV)	B vit. (0,+,++)
Knudsen, Cottage Doubles, apples & cinn.	1 cont	140	2	Na	1.5	0	15	Na	15	0	0
Knudsen, Cottage Doubles, pineapple	1 cont	130	2.5	Na	1.5	0	14	Na	8	0	0
Organic Valley, small curd	½ c	100	2	Na	1.5	0	<1	0	6	0	0
Cream Cheese (Philadelphia brand)											
Blueberry	1.2 oz	90	7	Na	4.5	0	5	0	2	0	0
Fat-free	1 oz	30	0	0	0	0	1	0	15	0	0
Garden vegetable	1.2 oz	90	8	Na	5	0	2	0	2	0	0
Original	1 oz	100	10	3	6	0	1	24*	0	0	0
Peaches 'n' cream	1.2 oz	90	7	Na	5	0	4	0	2	0	0
Salmon	1.2 oz	80	8	Na	4.5	0	1	0	2	0	0
Whipped	¾ oz	60	6	Na	3.5	0	1	0	0	0	0
Whipped, chives	¾ oz	60	6	Na	3.5	0	1	0	0	0	0
Whipped, mixed berry	¾ oz	60	6	Na	3.5	0	3	0	0	0	0
Edam (generic)	1 oz	99	8	2	5	0	0	3	20	0	0
Feta crumbles (Organic Valley)	1 oz	60	4	Na	2.5	0	0	Na	10	0	0
Gorgonzola crumbles (Athenos)	3 tbs	110	9	Na	6	1	0	3	15	0	0
Gouda (generic)	1 oz	99	8	2	5	0	1	3	19	0	0
Monterey Jack (generic)	1 oz	104	8	2.5	5	0	0	21	20	0	0
Monterey Jack, reduced fat, shredded (Organic Valley)	¼ c	80	5	Na	3.5	0	0	0	20	0	0
Mozzarella, singles 2% (Kraft)	1 slice	50	2.5	Na	1.5	0	2	Na	20	0	0
Mozzarella, string part skim (Organic Valley)	1 oz	81	5	Na	3	0	0	11*	20	0	0
Mozzarella, part skim shredded (Organic Valley)	¼ c	60	5	Na	3	0	0	0	20	0	0

Food	Portion Size	Calories	Total Fat (g)	Good Fats (g)	Bad Fats (g)	Fiber (g)	Sugars (mg)	Beta-carotene (mcg)	Calcium (%DV)	Vit. C (%DV)	B vit. (0,+,++)
Mozzarella, fat free, shredded (Polly-O)	1 oz	40	0	0	0	0	1	11*	15	0	0
Mozzarella, part skim (Polly-O)	1 oz	70	5	Na	3	0	1	11*	10	0	0
Muenster (Organic Valley)	1 oz	100	8	Na	5	0	0	0	20	0	0
Parmesan, shredded (Organic Valley)	1 oz	110	7	Na	4	0	0	0	35	0	0
Parmesan, grated (Polly-O)	5 g	20	1.5	Na	1	0	0	1*	6	0	0
Provolone (Organic Valley)	1 oz	100	8	Na	5	0	0	0	20	0	0
Ricotta, part skim (Polly-O)	¼ c	90	6	Na	4	0	2	5*	25	0	0
Swiss, singles 2% (Kraft)	1 slice	50	2.5	Na	1.5	0	1	19*	25	0	0
Swiss, deli style (Sargento)	1 slice	110	8	Na	4.5	0	0	19*	30	0	0
CHEESE SUBSTITUTES											
Better Than Cream Cheese, plain (Tofutti)	2 tbs	80	8	Na	2	0	0	0	Na	Na	Na
Soy American (Tofutti)	1 slice	70	5	Na	2	0	0	0	Na	Na	Na
Soy cheddar, Veggie shreds (Galaxy)	1 oz	70	4	2.5	0	0	0	0	30	4	+
Soy mozzarella, slices (Tofutti)	1 slice	70	5	Na	3	0	0	0	Na	Na	Na
Soy parmesan (Galaxy), grated	2 tsp	15	0.5	0	0	0	0	0	6	0	0
CHEESE SPREADS											
Kraft, Cheese Whiz, light	2 tbs	80	3.5	0	2	0	4	0	15	0	0
Kraft, Cheese Whiz, original	2 tbs	90	6	0	4.5	0	3	0	10	0	0
Kraft, pimento & olive spread	2 tbs	70	6	0	4	0	2	0	0	0	0
Kraft, roca blue	2 tbs	80	7	0	4.5	0	1	0	0	0	0
Velveeta, light	2 tbs	60	3	0	2	0	2	0	16	0	0
Velveeta, Mexican mild	2 tbs	90	6	0	4	0	2	0	0	0	0
Velveeta, original	2 tbs	80	6	0	4	0	2	0	15	0	0

Food	Portion Size	Calories	Total Fat (g)	Good Fats (g)	Bad Fats (g)	Fiber (g)	Sugars (mg)	Beta-carotene (mcg)	Calcium (%DV)	Vit. C (%DV)	B vit. (B,+,++)
CHERRIES											
Raw, sour, red, pitted	1 c	77	0	0	0	2	13	1193	2	25	0
Raw, sweet, red, pitted	1 c	91	0	0	0	3	19	55	1	16	0
Canned, dark sweet (Del Monte)	½ c	100	0	0	0	<1	24	115*	0	6	0
Canned, dark sweet (S&W)	½ c	140	0	0	0	1	26	115*	0	2	0
Frozen (Dole)	1 c	90	0	0	0	3	18	292*	0	2	0
CHERRY BEVERAGES											
Knudsen, black cherry spritzer	12 oz	180	0	0	0	0	39	Na	4	0	0
Knudsen, cherry cider	8 oz	130	0	0	0	0	30	Na	2	0	0
Knudsen, just black cherry	8 oz	180	0	0	0	0	24	Na	2	0	0
Minute Maid Cooler, clear cherry, pouch	200 mL	100	0	0	0	0	27	Na	10	100	0
CHESTNUTS											
Chinese, roasted	1 oz	68	0	0	0	0	0	0	0	17	0
European, roasted	1 oz	69	1	0	0	1	3	3	0	12	0
Japanese, roasted	1 oz	57	0	0	0	0	0	0	0	13	0
CHICKEN, fresh, broiler or fryer											
Breast & skin, roasted	4 oz	224	8	3	4	0	0	0	1	0	+
Breast only, roasted	4 oz	188	4	1	0	0	0	0	1	0	+
Dark & skin, roasted	4 oz	284	16	6	4	0	0	0	1	0	+
Dark only, roasted	4 oz	232	12	3.5	4	0	0	0	1	0	+
Drumstick, no skin, fried	1	82	3	1	1	0	0	0	0	0	+
Leg, no skin, fried	1	196	9	3	2	0	0	0	1	0	+
Light meat, no skin, fried	1 c	269	8	3	2	0	0	0	2	0	‡
Thigh, no skin, fried	1	113	5	2	1	0	0	0	0	0	+

Food	Portion Size	Calories	Total Fat (g)	Good Fats (g)	Bad Fats (g)	Fiber (g)	Sugars (mg)	Beta-carotene (mcg)	Calcium (%DV)	Vit. C (%DV)	B vit. (0,+,++)
CHICKEN, other											
Capon, meat & skin, roasted	4 oz	260	12	4.5	4	0	0	0	0	0	+
Cornish game hen, roasted	1 bird	245	9	3	2	0	0	0	2	2	‡‡
Giblets, simmered	1 c	281	13	2	4	0	0	0	1	15	‡‡
Liver, simmered	4 oz	188	8	1.5	4	0	0	30	1	46	‡‡
CHICKEN, refrigerated or frozen											
Breast, boneless, skinless (Organic Valley)	4 oz	120	1.5	0	0	0	0	0	0	2	+
Breast nuggets, cooked (Organic Valley)	5 pcs	200	12	Na	3.5	0	2	0	6	0	+
Breast tenderloins (Perdue											
Tender & Tasty)	4 oz	110	2	Na	0	0	1	0	0	2	++
Ground, frozen (Organic Valley)	4 oz	200	12	Na	3	0	0	0	2	0	+
Tyson											
Breast fillet Thin & Fancy	4 oz	120	1	0	0	0	0	0	0	0	+
Breast fillet, mesquite, bagged	1 pc	130	7	Na	2	0	0	0	0	0	+
Breast strips, boxed	3 oz	120	3.5	1.5	1	0	0	0	0	0	+
Chicken Bites	3 oz	270	18	7	4	1	0	0	0	0	+
Nuggets, frozen, bagged	5 pcs	280	18	7	4	0	0	0	0	0	+
Strips, buffalo style	2 pcs	230	10	3.5	2	1	0	0	0	0	+
Strips, crispy chicken	2 pcs	200	10	3.5	2	1	0	0	0	0	+
Tenders, honey battered, boxed	5 pcs	220	13	5	3	2	3	0	0	0	+
Wings, hot 'n spicy	3 pcs	219	15	6	3.5	0	0	0	0	0	+
Weaver											
Breast strips	3 pcs	230	14	Na	3.5	1	1	0	0	0	++
Breast tenders	5 pcs	240	14	Na	3	0	0	0	0	0	++

Food	Portion Size	Calories	Total Fat (g)	Good Fats (g)	Bad Fats (g)	Fiber (g)	Sugars (mg)	Beta-carotene (mcg)	Calcium (%DV)	Vit. C (%DV)	B vit. (0,+,++)
Buffalo popcorn chicken	7 pcs	230	14	Na	2	1	1	0	0	0	+
Crispy mini-drums	5 pcs	250	16	Na	3.5	1	2	0	2	0	+
Italian style patties	1	210	14	Na	3	1	1	0	6	0	+
Nuggets	4	230	15	Na	3.5	1	0	0	0	0	+
Original patties	1	180	11	Na	2.5	1	1	0	6	0	+
CHICKEN SUBSTITUTES											
Morningstar Farms											
Buffalo wings	5 wings	200	9	2.5	1.5	3	1	0	2	0	+
Chik 'n Nuggets	4 pcs	190	7	2	1	2	1	0	2	0	+
Chik 'n Patties, parmesan ranch	1	170	7	2	1	2	1	0	2	0	+
Chik 'n Tenders	2 pcs	190	7	2	1	3	1	0	4	0	+
Worthington											
Diced Chik, fat free	1/4 c	50	0	0	0	1	0	0	0	0	+
Fried Chik 'n gravy	2 pcs	150	10	2.5	1.5	2	0	0	2	0	++
Meatless chicken roll	3/8" slice	90	4.5	1	0.5	1	0	0	10	0	+
Meatless chicken slices	3 slices	90	4.5	1	1	<1	0	0	25	0	+
CHICKPEAS (garbanzo beans)											
Eden, organic	1/2 c	130	1	0	0	5	<1	0	6	0	+
Progresso	1/2 c	100	1.5	Na	0	4	2	0	2	0	+
S&W	1/2 c	80	1	0	0	5	2	0	2	2	
CHILI & CHILI BEANS											
Chili w/beans, canned	1 c	286	14	6	6	11	3	463	12	7	++
Chili beans, ranch style, canned	1 c	245	3	0	0.5	11	11	17	7	7	++

Food	Portion Size	Calories	Total Fat (g)	Good Fats (g)	Bad Fats (g)	Fiber (g)	Sugars (mg)	Beta-carotene (mcg)	Calcium (%DV)	Vit. C (%DV)	B vit. (0,+,++)
Eden, chili beans w/jalapeno & red pepper	½ c	130	0	0	0	7	1	0	6	0	+
Fantastic Foods, vegetarian chili	1 c	200	2	Na	0	7	7	0	10	35	Na
S&W, Santa Fe chili beans	1 c	160	0	0	0	6	4	0	4	8	0
S&W, chili beans w/tomato sauce	½ c	110	1	0	0	6	4	0	6	6	0
Stagg, Classic Chili	1 c	330	17	7	8	5	7	0	6	2	0
Stagg, Country Brand	1 c	320	16	7.5	7	5	6	0	4	2	0
Stagg, Laredo	1 c	320	15	Na	7	5	13	0	4	2	0
Stagg, Ranch House chicken chili	1 c	240	8	4	2	7	5	0	6	0	0
Stagg, Turkey Ranchero	1 c	240	3	0.5	1	6	6	0	6	6	0
Stagg, Vegetable Garden 4-bean	1 c	200	1	0	0	8	9	0	6	2	0
CHOCOLATE, baking											
Baker's baking unsweetened squares	½ oz	70	7	2	4.5	5	0	0	2	0	0
Baker's bittersweet squares	½ oz	70	6	Na	3	1	5	0	0	0	0
Baker's chocolate chunks semi-sweet	½ oz	70	4.5	1	2.5	1	8	0	0	0	0
Baker's German sweet	½ oz	60	3.5	Na	2	1	8	0	0	0	0
Baker's Premium white squares	½ oz	80	4.5	Na	3	0	8	0	2	0	0
CLAMS											
Bumble Bee, canned, chopped	¼ c	25	0	0	0	0	0	0	0	0	+
Bumble Bee, whole baby	¼ c	50	0	0	0	0	0	0	0	0	++
Chicken of the Sea, chopped	¼ c	30	0	0	0	0	0	0	0	0	++
COCONUT											
Fresh, raw, shredded	1 c	283	27	1	24	7	5	0	1	4	0
Baker's Angel Flake, shredded, sweetened	2 oz	70	5	Na	4.5	1	5	0	0	0	0

111

Food	Portion Size	Calories	Total Fat (g)	Good Fats (g)	Bad Fats (g)	Fiber (g)	Sugars (mg)	Beta-carotene (mcg)	Calcium (%DV)	Vit. C (%DV)	B vit. (0,+,++)
COD											
Atlantic, baked	3 oz	89	1	0	0	0	0	0	1	1	+
Atlantic, canned	3 oz	89	1	0	0	0	0	0	1	1	+
Pacific, baked	3 oz	88	1	0	0	0	0	0	0	4	+
COFFEE, flavored											
General Foods Int'l											
Café Francais	1 serv	60	3.5	Na	2.5	0	4	0	0	0	0
French vanilla	1 serv	60	2/5	Na	0.5	0	8	0	0	0	0
French vanilla, sugar free	1 serv	30	2.5	Na	2	0	0	0	0	0	0
Italian cappuccino	1 serv	50	1.5	0	1.5	0	8	0	0	0	0
Suisse mocha	1 serv	60	2	Na	1.5	0	9	0	0	0	0
Viennese chocolate	1 serv	50	1.5	0	1.5	0	9	0	0	0	+
COLLARDS, fresh, cooked, no salt	1 c	49	1	0	0	5	1	9146	26	57	+
COOKIES, mixes & unbaked											
Betty Crocker											
Chocolate Chip, pouch	2 cookie	120	3	Na	1.5	0	14	0	0	0	0
Oatmeal, pouch	2 cookie	110	1.5	Na	0	<1	11	0	0	0	0
Peanut butter, pouch	2 cookie	120	4	Na	1	0	12	0	0	0	0
Sugar, pouch	2 cookie	120	2.5	Na	0.5	0	13	0	0	0	0
Pillsbury											
Big Deluxe Classic, peanut butter cup	1 cookie	190	9	Na	5	1	15	0	0	0	0
Big Deluxe Classic, turtle supreme	1 cookie	200	10	Na	5	1	17	0	0	0	0
Chocolate chip, Create 'n Bake	1 oz	120	5	Na	2.5	<1	11	0	0	0	0
Oatmeal chocolate chip, Create 'n Bake	1 oz	130	6	Na	3.5	<1	10	0	0	0	0

Food	Portion Size	Calories	Total Fat (g)	Good Fats (g)	Bad Fats (g)	Fiber (g)	Sugars (mg)	Beta-carotene (mcg)	Calcium (%DV)	Vit. C (%DV)	B vit. (0,+,++)
Ready to Bake chocolate candy	1 cookie	100	5	Na	2.5	0	9	0	0	0	0
Ready to Bake chocolate chunk & chip	1 cookie	100	5	Na	2.5	0	8	0	0	0	0
Ready to Bake sugar	1 cookie	5	Na	3	0	7	0	0	0	0	0
COOKIES, ready-to-eat											
Barbara's Bakery											
Fig bar, apple cinnamon	1	60	0	0	0	1	9	0	0	2	0
Fig bar, blueberry	1	70	0.5	0	0	0	9	0	0	2	0
Fig bar, traditional	1	60	0.5	0	0	1	8	0	0	8	0
Fig bar, whole wheat	1	60	0	0	0	1	8	0	0	8	0
Ginger organic mini cookies	1 pkg	100	2	Na	1	0	8	0	0	0	0
Snackimals, chocolate chip	10 pcs	120	4	Na	0	0	8	0	0	0	0
Snackimals, vanilla	10 pcs	110	4	Na	0	0	5	0	4	0	0
Snackimals, wheat-free	10 pcs	120	5	Na	0	1	6	0	4	0	0
Famous Amos											
Chocolate chip & pecans	4 pcs	150	8	Na	4	<1	10	0	0	0	0
Chocolate crème sandwich	3 pcs	160	6	Na	4	<1	14	0	0	0	0
Iced gingersnaps, low fat	2 oz pkg	200	3	Na	1.5	1	17	0	0	0	0
Oatmeal chocolate chip walnut	4 pcs	140	7	Na	4	1	9	0	0	0	0
Keebler											
Animal cookies, frosted	8 cookie	150	7	Na	5	1	13	0	0	0	0
Chip Deluxe, chocolate lovers	1 cookie	80	4.5	Na	3	0	5	0	0	0	0
Chips Deluxe coconut	1 cookie	80	4.5	Na	3.5	1	4	0	0	0	0
Chips Deluxe, peanut butter cups	1 cookie	90	4.5	Na	3.5	0	5	0	0	0	0
EL Fudge double stuffed	2 cookie	180	9	Na	5.5	1	14	0	0	0	0

Food	Portion Size	Calories	Total Fat (g)	Good Fats (g)	Bad Fats (g)	Fiber (g)	Sugars (mg)	Beta-carotene (mcg)	Calcium (%DV)	Vit. C (%DV)	B vit. (0,+,++)
Fudge Shoppe, deluxe graham	3 cookie	140	7	Na	6	1	10	0	0	0	0
Fudge Shoppe, filled peanut butter	2 cookie	170	11	Na	5.5	<1	19	0	0	0	0
Fudge Shoppe, fudge sticks	3 cookie	150	8	Na	6.5	0	15	0	0	0	0
Golden vanilla wafers	8 cookie	140	6	Na	3.5	<1	9	0	0	0	0
Oatmeal, country style	2 cookie	130	6	Na	4	1	8	0	0	0	0
Sandies, chocolate chip pecan	1 cookie	80	5	Na	3	0	4	0	0	0	0
Sandies, fruit delights, strawberry cheesecake	1 cookie	80	3.5	Na	2	0	6	0	0	0	0
Sandies, pecan	1 cookie	80	5	Na	3.5	0	3	0	0	0	0
Sandies, pecan, reduced fat	1 cookie	80	3.5	Na	2	0	4	0	0	0	0
Sandies, simply shortbread	1 cookie	80	4.5	Na	4	0	4	0	0	0	0
Sandies, swirl cinnamon	1 cookie	90	5	Na	3.5	<1	3	0	0	0	0
Soft Batch, chocolate chip	1 cookie	80	3.5	Na	2	<1	6	0	0	0	0
Soft Batch, oatmeal raisin	1 cookie	80	3	Na	1.5	<1	6	0	0	0	0
Vienna Fingers	2 cookie	150	7	Na	5	<1	10	0	0	0	0
Vienna Fingers, reduced fat	2 cookie	140	5	Na	3.5	<1	11	0	0	0	0
Murray Sugar Free											
Chocolate chip	3 cookie	140	8	Na	5	1	0	0	0	0	0
Chocolate sandwich cream	3 cookie	130	7	Na	4	1	0	0	0	0	0
Double fudge	3 cookie	140	7	Na	4	2	0	0	0	0	0
Lemon wafers	4 cookie	140	8	Na	5	5	0	0	0	0	0
Peanut butter	3 cookie	160	10	Na	4.5	1	0	0	0	0	0
Shortbread	8 cookie	130	5	Na	3	1	0	0	0	0	0
Shortbread, pecan	3 cookie	170	11	Na	6	1	0	0	0	0	0
Vanilla wafers	9 cookie	130	5	Na	3	1	0	0	0	0	0

Nabisco

Food	Portion Size	Calories	Total Fat (g)	Good Fats (g)	Bad Fats (g)	Fiber (g)	Sugars (mg)	Beta-carotene (mcg)	Calcium (%DV)	Vit. C (%DV)	B vit. (0,+,++)
Chips Ahoy, 100% whole grain	1 cookie	150	Na	2.5	2	10	0	0	0	0	0
Chips Ahoy, chunky white fudge	1 cookie	80	4	Na	1.5	1	6	0	0	0	0
Chips Ahoy, chunky chocolate chip	1 cookie	80	4	Na	1.5	1	6	0	0	0	0
Chips Ahoy, reduced fat	1 cookie	140	5	Na	2	1	11	0	2	0	0
Nilla Wafers	1 oz	140	6	Na	1.5	0	11	0	2	0	0
Nilla Wafers, reduced fat	1 oz	120	2	Na	0	0	12	0	2	0	0
Nutter Butter sandwich	2 cookie	130	5	Na	1.5	1	8	0	0	0	0
Oreo sandwich	3 cookie	160	7	Na	2	1	14	0	0	0	0
Oreo sandwich, Double Stuf	2 cookie	140	7	Na	2.5	1	13	0	0	0	0
Oreo sandwich, reduced fat	3 cookie	150	4.5	Na	1	1	14	0	0	0	0
Pepperidge Farm											
Bordeaux	4 cookie	130	5	Na	3.5	1	12	0	0	0	0
Brussels	3 cookie	150	7	Na	4	1	11	0	0	0	0
Chocolate chunk milk choc, macadamia	1 cookie	140	8	Na	3.5	0	9	0	0	0	0
Double chocolate chunk, dark chocolate	1 cookie	140	7	Na	3	1	10	0	0	0	0
Milano, original	3 cookie	180	10	Na	5	1	11	0	0	0	0
Shortbread	2 cookie	140	7	Na	4	1	5	0	0	0	0
Soft Bake, sugar	1 cookie	140	5	Na	2.5	0	11	0	0	0	0
CORN											
Fresh, cooked, white or yellow, no salt	1 c	177	2	0.5	2	4	5	80	0	17	+
Fresh, cooked, white or yellow, cob	7" cob	77	1	0	0	2	3	46	0	10	+

Food	Portion Size	Calories	Total Fat (g)	Good Fats (g)	Bad Fats (g)	Fiber (g)	Sugars (mg)	Beta-carotene (mcg)	Calcium (%DV)	Vit. C (%DV)	B vit. (0,+,++)
Canned											
Del Monte, Savory Sides, in butter sauce	1/2 c	90	2.5	Na	1	<1	5	50*	0	8	+
Del Monte, Savory Sides, Fiesta corn	1/2 c	50	1	0	0	2	5	Na	0	6	0
Del Monte, Savory Sides, gold & white	1/2 c	80	0.5	0	0	2	6	34*	0	6	0
Del Monte, Savory Sides, Santa Fe	1/2 c	70	1	0	0	1	1	34*	0	15	0
Del Monte, Savory Sides, white, cream	1/2 c	100	1	0	0	2	6	0	0	4	0
Green Giant, creamed corn	1/2 c	90	0.5	0	0	1	7	38	0	2	+
Green Giant, extra sweet niblets	1/3 c	50	0.5	0	0	1	4	18*	0	2	0
Green Giant, Mexicorn	1/3 c	70	0.5	0	0	1	4	0	0	6	+
Green Giant, whole kernel sweet	1/2 c	80	0.5	0	0	1	6	20*	0	4	0
S&W, creamed corn	1/2 c	60	0.5	0	0	2	7	38*	0	4	0
S&W, whole kernels	1/2 c	60	1	0	0	3	7	25*	0	6	0
Frozen											
Bird's Eye, baby gold & white	2/3 c	100	1	0	0	2	3	Na	0	8	0
Bird's Eye, baby white corn kernels	2/3 c	100	1	0	0	3	3	Na	0	10	0
Cascadian Farms, organic sweet	3/4 c	90	1	0	0	2	4	Na	0	6	0
Green Giant, cream style	1/2 c	110	1	0	0	2	7	0	0	6	0
Green Giant, niblets w/butter	2/3 c	110	2	Na	1	2	5	40*	0	4	0
Green Giant, shoepeg white, no sauce	3/4 c	100	1.5	0.5	0	2	3	0	0	4	0
CORN CHIPS											
Bugles, chili cheese	1 1/3 c	160	9	0.5	7	.5	2	0	0	0	0
Bugles, original	1 1/3 c	160	9	0.5	8	<1	1	0	0	0	0
Bugles, salsa	1 1/3 c	160	9	Na	7	<1	2	0	0	0	0
Bugles, smokin' BBQ	1 1/3 c	150	8	Na	7	0	3	0	0	0	0

116

Food	Portion Size	Calories	Total Fat (g)	Good Fats (g)	Bad Fats (g)	Fiber (g)	Sugars (mg)	Beta-carotene (mcg)	Calcium (%DV)	Vit. C (%DV)	B vit. (0,+,++)
Doritos, cool ranch tortilla	1 oz	140	7	4*	1	1	<1	0	2	0	0
Doritos, light nacho cheese	1 oz	100	2	Na	0.5	2	<1	0	2	0	0
Doritos, nacho cheese tortilla	1 oz	140	8	4*	1.5	1	1	0	2	0	0
Doritos, nacho cheese tortilla, baked	1 oz	120	3.5	1	0.5	1	1	0	4	0	0
Doritos, ranchero tortilla	1 oz	140	7	4	1	1	1	0	2	6	0
Doritos, toasted corn	1 oz	140	7	Na	1	1	0	0	4	0	0
Fritos, bar-b-q	1 oz	150	10	Na	1.5	1	<1	0	4	0	0
Fritos, cheese flavor	1 oz	160	10	Na	1.5	1	<1	0	4	0	0
Fritos, flamin' hot	1 oz	160	10	Na	1.5	1	<1	0	4	0	0
Fritos, original	1 oz	160	10	Na	1.5	1	<1	0	2	0	0
Herrs, bite size dippers	1 oz	140	6	Na	1.5	2	0	0	0	0	0
Herrs, corn chips	1 oz	160	10	Na	2	2	0	0	0	0	0
Herrs, nachitos	1 oz	140	6	Na	1	2	0	0	0	0	0
Tostitos, restaurant style tortilla	1 oz	140	7	Na	1	2	0	0	4	0	0
Tostitos, sensations red chile & lime	1 oz	150	8	Na	1	2	0	0	2	0	0
COUSCOUS											
Fantastic Foods											
Organic, dry	1/4 c	150	0.5	0	0	1	1	0	0	0	+
Organic, whole wheat, uncooked	1/4 c	170	0.5	0	0	6	1	0	2	0	+
Near East											
Herb chicken, mix	2 oz	190	1	0	0	2	2	0	2	0	+
Mediterranean curry, mix	2 oz	190	1	0	0	3	2	0	2	2	++
Original plain, mix	2 oz	220	1	0	0	2	1	0	0	0	+++

Food	Portion Size	Calories	Total Fat (g)	Good Fats (g)	Bad Fats (g)	Fiber (g)	Sugars (mg)	Beta-carotene (mcg)	Calcium (%DV)	Vit. C (%DV)	B vit. (0,+,++)
Parmesan, mix	2 oz	200	2	0	0.5	3	3	0	2	4	+
Toasted pine nut, mix	2 oz	200	3	0	0.5	2	2	0	2	0	+
CRAB											
Bumble Bee, canned, white	¼ c	40	1	0	0	0	0	0	2	0	0
Bumble Bee, pink, canned	¼ c	35	0.5	0	0	0	0	Na	2	0	0
Fresh, cooked, blue	1 c	120	2	0	0	0	0	0	2	6	‡
Fresh, cooked, Dungeness	3 oz	93	1	0	0	0	0	0	5	5	‡
CRACKERS											
Eden Foods, brown rice	8 pcs	120	2	0	0	2	1	0	2	0	0
Eden Foods, nori maki rice	15 pcs	110	0	0	0	2	<1	0	4	0	0
Keebler											
Club, original	4 pcs	70	3	1	1	<1	1	0	0	0	0
Club, reduced fat	5 pcs	70	2.5	1	0.5	<1	2	0	0	0	0
Grahams, cinnamon crisp	8 pcs	130	3.5	1.5	1	1	9	0	10	0	0
Grahams, cinnamon crisp, low-fat	8 pcs	110	1.5	0.5	0	1	9	0	10	0	0
Grahams, honey	8 pcs	140	4	1.5	1	<1	7	0	10	0	0
Grahams, original	8 pcs	130	3.5	1.5	1	<1	7	0	10	0	0
Scooby-Doo graham cracker sticks	9 pcs	130	4	Na	0.5	<1	8	0	10	0	0
Scooby-Doo graham cracker sticks, honey	9 pcs	130	4	Na	0.5	<1	8	0	10	0	0
Sunshine, Cheez-it, fiesta cheddar nacho	25 pcs	160	8	Na	2.5	<1	10	0	2	0	0
Sunshine, Cheez-it, hot & spicy	25 pcs	150	8	Na	2	<1	0	0	0	0	0
Sunshine, Cheez-it, original	27 pcs	160	8	Na	2	<1	<1	0	4	0	0
Sunshine, Cheez-it, Twisterz cool ranch	17 pcs	140	6	Na	2.5	<1	1	0	0	0	0
Sunshine, Cheez-it, white cheddar	25 pcs	150	8	Na	2.5	<1	0	0	0	0	0

Food	Portion Size	Calories	Total Fat (g)	Good Fats (g)	Bad Fats (g)	Fiber (g)	Sugars (mg)	Beta-carotene (mcg)	Calcium (%DV)	Vit. C (%DV)	B vit. (0,+,++)
Toasteds, Buttercrisp	5 pcs	80	3.5	1.5	1	<1	1	0	0	0	0
Toasteds, onion	5 pcs	80	3.5	1.5	1	<1	2	0	0	0	0
Toasteds, sesame	5 pcs	80	3.5	1.5	1	<1	1	0	0	0	0
Toasteds, wheat	5 pcs	80	3.5	1.5	1	<1	1	0	0	0	0
Townhouse Bistro, multigrain	2 pcs	80	3	Na	1.5	<1	2	0	0	0	0
Townhouse Bistro corn bread	2 pcs	80	3	Na	1.5	<1	1	0	0	0	0
Wheatables, honey wheat	17 pcs	140	6	2	1.5	1	4	0	0	0	0
Wheatables, originals	17 pcs	140	6	2.5	1.5	1	4	0	0	0	0
Wheatables, reduced fat	19 pcs	140	4	1.5	1	1	5	0	0	0	0
Zesta, original	5 pcs	60	1.5	0.5	1	<1	0	0	0	0	0
Zesta, whole grain wheat	5 pcs	60	1.5	0.5	1	<1	<1	0	0	0	0
Nabisco											
Cheese Nips, cheddar	1 oz	150	6	Na	1.5	1	0	0	2	0	0
Cheese Nips, four cheese	1 oz	150	7	Na	2	1	1	0	2	0	0
Ritz Bits, cracker sandwich, peanut butter	1 oz	140	8	Na	1.5	1	3	0	4	0	0
Ritz, Dinosaurs	1 oz	130	3	3	1	0	3	0	6	0	0
Ritz, original	½ oz	80	4.5	3	1	0	1	0	2	0	0
Ritz, reduced fat	½ oz	70	2	Na	0	0	1	0	2	0	0
Ritz, Top-ems	½ oz	70	3	Na	0.5	0	1	0	2	0	0
Ritz, whole wheat	½ oz	70	2.5	Na	0.5	1	1	0	2	0	0
Triscuit, deli-style rye	1 oz	120	4.5	Na	0.5	3	0	0	0	0	0
Triscuit, garden herb	1 oz	120	4	Na	0.5	3	0	0	0	0	0
Triscuit, original	1 oz	120	4.5	Na	0.5	3	0	0	0	0	0
Triscuit, reduced fat	1 oz	120	3	Na	0	3	0	0	0	0	0

Food	Portion Size	Calories	Total Fat (g)	Good Fats (g)	Bad Fats (g)	Fiber (g)	Sugars (mg)	Beta-carotene (mcg)	Calcium (%DV)	Vit. C (%DV)	B Vit. (0,+,++)
Wheat Thins, honey	1 oz	140	6	Na	1	1	5	0	2	0	0
Wheat Thins, multigrain	1 oz	130	4.5	Na	0.5	2	3	0	4	0	0
Wheat Thins, original	1 oz	160	7	2	1	1	4	0	2	0	0
Wheat Thins, ranch	1 oz	130	6	Na	1	1	4	0	2	0	0
Wheat Thins, reduced fat	1 oz	130	5	Na	0.5	1	3	0	2	0	0
Pepperidge Farm Goldfish											
Cheddar	89 pcs	140	5	Na	1	1	1	0	4	0	0
Parmesan	60 pcs	130	4	Na	1	1	1	0	6	0	0
Pizza	55 pcs	140	5	Na	1	1	1	0	2	0	0
Pretzel	43 pcs	130	2.5	Na	0.5	1	1	0	0	0	0
CRANBERRY											
Fresh, raw	1 c	51	0	0	0	4	4	34	0	21	0
Sauce, canned, whole berry (S&W)	1/4 c	100	0	0	0	1	17	16	0	0	0
Sauce, canned, jellied	1/4 c	100	0	0	0	1	17	16	0	0	0
CRANBERRY BEVERAGES											
Langers, cranberry juice cocktail	8 oz	140	0	0	0	0	32	Na	0	100	0
Langers, diet cranberry	8 oz	30	0	0	0	0	8	Na	20	100	0
Langers, white cranberry	8 oz	120	0	0	0	0	28	Na	0	100	0
Langers, white cranberry raspberry	8 oz	120	0	0	0	0	28	Na	0	100	0
Santa Cruz, cranberry nectar, organic	8 oz	110	0	0	0	0	26	Na	2	2	0
CREAM											
Half & half	1 oz	39	3	1	2	0	0	6	3	0	0
Half & half, fat-free	1 oz	18	0	0	0	0	2	1	2	0	0

Food	Portion Size	Calories	Total Fat (g)	Good Fats (g)	Bad Fats (g)	Fiber (g)	Sugars (mg)	Beta-carotene (mcg)	Calcium (%DV)	Vit. C (%DV)	B vit. (0,+,++)
Heavy whipping cream	1 oz	103	11	3	7	0	0	21	1	0	0
Light whipping cream	1 oz	83	9	1.5	5	0	0	18	0	0	0
CREAMERS (coffee)											
Coffee-Mate, liquid, amaretto	1 tbs	35	1.5	0	0	0	5	0	0	0	0
Coffee-Mate, liquid, chocolate raspberry	1 tbs	35	1.5	0	0	0	5	0	0	0	0
Coffee-Mate, powder, coconut cream	4 tsp	60	2.5	0	2	0	7	0	0	0	0
Coffee-Mate, powder, creamy chocolate	4 tsp	60	2.5	0	2	0	7	0	0	0	0
International Delight, amaretto	1 tbs	40	1.5	Na	1	0	6	0	0	0	0
International Delight, chocolate caramel	1 tbs	45	2	Na	1	0	6	0	0	0	0
International Delight, French vanilla	1 tbs	40	2	Na	1	0	6	0	0	0	0
CROUTONS											
Pepperidge Farm, Classic Caesar	6 pcs	35	1.5	Na	0	0	1	0	0	0	0
Pepperidge Farm, four cheese & garlic	6 pcs	30	1	Na	0	0	1	0	1	0	0
CUCUMBER, raw, sliced, peeled	1 c	14	0	0	0	1	2	37	1	6	0
CURRANTS, raw, red & white	1 c	63	0	0	0	5	8	28	3	76	+
Zante (Sun-Maid)	1/4 c	120	0	0	0	3	24	15*	3	3	0
DANDELION GREENS, cooked, chopped	1 c	35	1	0	0	3	3	6247	14	31	0
DATES, pitted, chopped	1 oz	80	0	0	0	2	15	2	0	0	0
Pitted (Dole)	1/4 c	120	0	0	0	3	28	Na	2	0	0
DESSERT TOPPINGS											
Cool Whip, French vanilla	9 g	25	1.5	0	1.5	0	1	0	0	0	0
Cool Whip, lite	9 g	20	1	0	1	0	1	0	0	0	0
Cool Whip, regular	9 g	25	1.5	0	1.5	0	1	0	0	0	0
Smucker's spoonable butterscotch	2 tbs	120	0	0	0	0	24	0	2	0	0

121

Food	Portion Size	Calories	Total Fat (g)	Good Fats (g)	Bad Fats (g)	Fiber (g)	Sugars (mg)	Beta-carotene (mcg)	Calcium (%DV)	Vit. C (%DV)	B vit. (0,+,++)
Smucker's Dove dark chocolate	2 tbs	130	4.5	Na	1.5	1	18	0	0	0	0
Smucker's sundae syrup, caramel	2 tbs	100	0	0	0	0	20	0	0	0	0
Smucker's sundae syrup, strawberry	2 tbs	110	0	0	0	0	23	0	0	0	0
Smucker's special recipe hot fudge	2 tbs	140	4	Na	1	<1	16	0	6	0	0
DIPS											
Kraft, creamy ranch	1 oz	60	4.5	Na	3	0	1	0	0	0	0
Kraft, French onion	1 oz	60	4.5	Na	3	0	1	0	0	0	0
Kraft, guacamole	1 oz	50	4.5	Na	2.5	0	1	0	0	0	0
Lay's, creamy ranch	2 tbs	60	5	Na	2.5	0	0	0	6	0	0
DUCK											
Roasted w/skin, diced	1 c	472	40	18	14	0	0	0	1	0	+
Roasted, without skin, diced	1 c	281	16	5	6	0	0	0	1	0	+
EGGS											
Chicken, whole, raw, large	1	73	5	2	2	0	0	5	2	0	+
Chicken, white only, large	1	17	0	0	0	0	0	0	0	0	0
Chicken, yolk only, large	1	55	5	2	2	0	0	15	2	0	0
Chicken, whole, hard boiled, large	1	77	5	2	2	0	0	5.5	2	0	0
Chicken, whole, poached, large	1	73	5	2	2	0	0	5	2	0	+
Duck, whole, fresh	1	129	10	4.5	3	0	1	10	4	0	+
Goose, whole, fresh	1	266	19	8	5	0	1	19	8	0	‡
Quail, whole, fresh	1	14	1	0	0	0	0	1	0	0	0
EGG SUBSTITUTES											
Ener-G-Egg	1½ tsp	15	0	0	0	0	0	0	0	0	0
Morningstar Scramblers	¼ c	35	0	0	0	0	0	Na	2	0	+

Food	Portion Size	Calories	Total Fat (g)	Good Fats (g)	Bad Fats (g)	Fiber (g)	Sugars (mg)	Beta-carotene (mcg)	Calcium (%DV)	Vit. C (%DV)	B vit. (0,+,++)
EGGPLANT, boiled, no salt, cubes	1 c	34	0	0	0	2	3	21	0	2	0
ENDIVE, raw, chopped	1 c	8	0	0	0	2	0	750	2	4	0
FAST FOOD, Arby's											
Arby's Melt sandwich	1	300	12	Na	5.5	1	5	Na	6	0	Na
Apple turnover, no icing	1	250	15	Na	10	2	15	0	1	3	0
Bacon biscuit	1	340	21	Na	6	1	3	0	3	0	Na
Bacon, beef & cheddar sandwich	1	520	27	Na	11	2	9	0	8	3	Na
Bacon & egg croissant	1	337	22	Na	10	1	3	0	4	2	Na
Beef & cheddar sandwich	1	440	21	Na	9	2	8	0	8	2	Na
Buttermilk ranch dressing	1 pkt	325	30	Na	6	0	2	0	4	1	0
Chicken breast fillet, crispy, sandwich	1	576	30	Na	6	3	11	0	17	9	Na
Chicken breast fillet, grilled, sandwich	1	410	17	Na	3	2	6	0	8	18	Na
Chicken tenders, 3 pack	1 pkt	379	18	Na	4	2	6	0	22	1	Na
Chicken tender, 5 pack	1 pkt	630	31	Na	7	3	0	0	37	2	Na
Chicken salad sandwich w/pecans	1	769	39	Na	10	1	17	0	8	50	Na
Corned beef reuben	1	606	33	Na	10	3	6	0	36	5	Na
Curly fries	Small	340	20	Na	6.5	4	0	0	4	8	Na
Curly fries	Medium	410	24	Na	8.5	5	0	0	5	10	Na
Curly fries	Large	630	37	Na	13	7	0	0	8	16	Na
Hot ham & swiss melt sandwich	1	275	6	Na	2	1	6	0	15	1	Na
Jalapeno bites, regular	5	275	6	Na	2	2	6	0	6	1	Na
Jr. roast beef sandwich	1	270	9	Na	4.5	1	5	0	5	0	Na
Kid's Meal, 2 pack chicken tenders	1 pkt	290	14	Na	3.5	1	0	0	17	1	Na
Loaded potato bites, small	5 pcs	353	22	Na	8	2	0	0	18	21	Na

Food	Portion Size	Calories	Total Fat (g)	Good Fats (g)	Bad Fats (g)	Fiber (g)	Sugars (mg)	Beta-carotene (mcg)	Calcium (%DV)	Vit. C (%DV)	B vit. (0,+,++)
Loaded potato bites, large	10 pcs	707	44	Na	17	5	0	0	37	41	Na
Mozzarella sticks, regular	4 pcs	426	28	Na	15	2	5	0	38	1	Na
Onion petals, regular	1	330	23	Na	5	2	7	0	2	1	Na
Roast beef, regular sandwich	1	320	14	Na	6	1	5	0	5	0	Na
Roast beef, medium sandwich	1	415	21	Na	10	2	5	0	6	0	Na
Roast beef, large sandwich	1	550	28	Na	14	3	6	0	7	0	Na
Roast turkey, ranch & bacon wrap	1	700	37	Na	12	3	4	0	1	14	Na
Salad: chicken club, no dressing	1	500	26	Na	10	5	4	0	38	60	Na
Salad: Martha's Vineyard, no dressing	1	270	8	Na	4	4	16	0	19	57	Na
Salad: Santa Fe, no dressing	1	500	23	Na	10	6	5	0	41	62	Na
Sausage biscuit	1	436	27	Na	9	1	3	0	3	0	Na
Sausage, egg & cheese wrap	1	688	45	Na	17	2	3	0	32	2	Na
Shake: chocolate, regular	1	510	13	Na	8	0	81	0	51	9	Na
Ultimate BLT sandwich	1	780	45	Na	12	6	18	0	16	28	Na
FAST FOOD, Baskin Robbins											
Black walnut	½ c	280	19	Na	9	1	23	0	15	2	0
Cherries jubilee	½ c	240	12	Na	7	1	26	0	15	2	0
Chocolate	½ c	260	14	Na	9	0	31	0	15	2	0
Chocolate almond	½ c	300	18	Na	9	1	29	0	15	2	0
Chocolate chip cookie dough	½ c	290	15	Na	10	1	30	0	15	2	0
Chocolate chip	½ c	270	16	Na	10	1	26	0	15	2	0
Chocolate oreo	½ c	330	19	Na	9	1	32	0	15	2	0
French vanilla	½ c	280	18	Na	11.5	0	25	0	15	2	0

124

Food	Portion Size	Calories	Total Fat (g)	Good Fats (g)	Bad Fats (g)	Fiber (g)	Sugars (mg)	Beta-carotene (mcg)	Calcium (%DV)	Vit. C (%DV)	B vit. (0,+,++)
Fudge brownie	½ c	300	19	Na	11	1	31	0	10	2	0
German chocolate cake	½ c	300	16	Na	9	1	35	0	15	2	0
Jamoca	½ c	240	13	Na	9	0	24	0	15	2	0
Mint chocolate chip	½ c	270	16	Na	10	1	26	0	15	2	0
Nutty coconut	½ c	300	20	Na	9	1	27	0	15	2	0
Oreo cookies cream	½ c	280	15	Na	9	1	27	0	15	2	0
Peanut butter & chocolate	½ c	320	20	Na	9	1	28	0	15	2	0
Pistachio almond	½ c	290	19	Na	9	1	23	0	15	2	0
Praline & cream	½ c	270	14	Na	8	0	33	0	15	2	0
Rocky road	½ c	290	15	Na	8	1	32	0	15	2	0
Vanilla	½ c	260	16	Na	10.5	0	26	0	15	2	0
Very berry strawberry	½ c	220	11	Na	7	0	27	0	15	20	0
Low-Fat, No Sugar Added Ice Cream											
Berries & bananas	½ c	110	2	Na	1	1	7	0	15	50	0
Blueberry swirl	½ c	130	2	Na	1	1	7	0	15	2	0
Caramel turtle	½ c	160	4	Na	3	0	7	0	15	2	0
Chocolate chip	½ c	170	4.5	Na	3.5	1	8	0	15	2	0
Tin roof sundae	½ c	190	3	Na	1.5	1	9	0	15	2	0
Sundaes											
2 scoop hot fudge sundae	1	530	29	Na	19	0	52	0	20	2	0
3 scoop hot fudge sundae	1	750	41	Na	27	0	74	0	30	4	0
Banana royale	1	630	27	Na	16	5	73	0	25	15	0
Banana split	1	1030	39	Na	23	7	140	0	35	30	0

Food	Portion Size	Calories	Total Fat (g)	Good Fats (g)	Bad Fats (g)	Fiber (g)	Sugars (mg)	Beta-carotene (mcg)	Calcium (%DV)	Vit. C (%DV)	B vit. (0,+,++)
Non-fat soft serve yogurt, no sugar added											
Butter pecan	½ c	90	0	0	0	1	6	0	15	2	0
Café mocha	½ c	90	0	0	0	1	7	0	15	2	0
Chocolate	½ c	80	0	0	0	1	6	0	15	2	0
Strawberry patch	½ c	90	0	0	0	1	6	0	15	2	0
Vanilla	½ c	90	0	0	0	1	6	0	15	2	0
Sherbet											
Blue raspberry	½ c	160	2	Na	1.5	0	34	0	4	2	0
Rock & pop	½ c	190	4	Na	3	0	36	0	4	0	0
Twisted chip	½ c	180	3	Na	1	0	36	0	4	4	0
Wild & reckless spirit	½ c	160	2	Na	1.5	0	33	0	6	0	0
FAST FOOD, Burger King											
BK Big fish sandwich	1	630	30	Na	8.5	4	8	0	10	2	Na
BK Big fish sandwich, w/o tartar sauce	1	470	13	Na	5	3	7	0	10	0	Na
BK Chicken fries	9 pcs	470	31	Na	10.5	3	2	0	2	0	Na
BK Veggie burger	1	420	4.5	Na	2.5	7	8	0	15	10	Na
Chicken tenders	8 pcs	340	20	Na	8	<1	<1	0	2	0	Na
Croisan'wich w/ham, egg, cheese	1	340	18	Na	8	<1	6	0	15	0	Na
Double Croisan'wich w/double sausage	1	680	51	Na	21	<1	6	0	25	0	Na
Double Whopper	1	900	57	Na	21	3	11	0	15	15	Na
Double Whopper w/cheese	1	990	64	Na	26.5	3	11	0	30	15	Na
Dutch apple pie	1	300	13	Na	6	1	23	0	0	0	Na
Enormous omelet sandwich	1	730	46	Na	18	0	<1	0	30	0	Na
French fries	Medium	360	20	Na	9	4	1	0	2	15	+*

Food	Portion Size	Calories	Total Fat (g)	Good Fats (g)	Bad Fats (g)	Fiber (g)	Sugars (mg)	Beta-carotene (mcg)	Calcium (%DV)	Vit. C (%DV)	B vit. (0,+,++)
French toast sticks	5	390	20	10*	9	2	11	0	6	0	Na
Garden salad, side	1	15	0	0	0	1	<1	Na	2	10	0
Hash browns	1 serv	230	15	na	9	2	0	0	0	2	Na
Onion rings	Medium	320	16	Na	7.5	3	5	0	10	6	Na
Shake, strawberry	Medium	660	19	Na	12	0	109	0	45	6	Na
Shake, vanilla	Medium	560	21	Na	13.5	0	77	0	50	6	Na
Tendercrisp chicken sandwich	1	780	43	Na	12	2	2	0	2	2	Na
Tendercrisp garden salad	1	400	21	Na	8.5	5	5	0	20	65	Na
Tendergrill chicken sandwich	1	450	10	Na	2	4	9	0	8	10	Na
Triple Whopper sandwich	1	1130	74	Na	30	3	11	0	15	15	Na
Triple Whopper sandwich w/cheese	1	1230	82	Na	35.5	3	11	0	30	15	Na
Whopper sandwich	1	670	39	Na	12.5	3	11	0	15	15	Na
Whopper jr sandwich	1	370	21	Na	6.5	2	6	0	8	6	Na
Whopper jr sandwich w/cheese	1	410	24	Na	9	2	6	0	15	6	Na
FAST FOOD, Church's Chicken											
Apple pie	1	260	11	Na	6	1	15	0	0	8	0
Cajun rice, regular	Regular	130	7	Na	3	<1	0	0	0	0	+*
Chicken fried steak sandwich	1	490	32	Na	10	2	4	0	0	2	Na
Chicken fried steak w/gravy	2 pcs	610	43	Na	17	2	7	0	4	0	Na
Cole slaw	Regular	150	10	Na	2	2	7	0	2	20	Na
Double lemon pie	1	300	14	Na	6	0	29	0	10	0	Na
French fries	Regular	420	20	Na	12	6	<1	0	4	2	+*
Jalapeno bombers	4	240	10	Na	6	3	5	0	20	0	Na
Macaroni & cheese	Regular	210	11	Na	4	1	6	0	12	0	Na

Food	Portion Size	Calories	Total Fat (g)	Good Fats (g)	Bad Fats (g)	Fiber (g)	Sugars (mg)	Beta-carotene (mcg)	Calcium (%DV)	Vit. C (%DV)	B vit. (0,+,++)
Okra	Regular	300	23	Na	4	6	1	0	11	3	Na
Original breast	1	200	11	Na	5	1	0	0	0	0	+*
Original leg	1	110	6	Na	3	0	0	0	0	0	+*
Original tender strip	1 pc	120	6	Na	3	<0.5	1	0	0	2	Na
Original thigh	1	330	23	Na	9	1	0	0	2	0	+*
Original wing	1	300	19	Na	8	3	0	0	2	2	+*
Spicy chicken sandwich	1	360	18	Na	5.5	3	3	0	8	2	+*
Spicy fish sandwich	1	320	20	Na	7	2	3	0	4	0	+*
Spicy tender strips	1 pc	135	7	Na	4	4	0	0	0	2	Na
Strawberry cream cheese pie	1 pie	280	15	Na	8	2	22	0	4	0	Na
FAST FOOD, Dairy Queen											
Desserts, Beverages											
Blizzard, banana split	Small	460	14	Na	9	<1	63	0	35	8	Na
Blizzard, banana split	Medium	580	17	Na	11.5	1	83	0	40	15	Na
Blizzard, banana split	Large	810	23	Na	16	2	115	0	60	20	Na
Blizzard, chocolate chip cookie dough	Small	720	28	Na	16.5	0	78	0	35	2	Na
Blizzard, chocolate chip cookie dough	Large	1320	52	Na	31	0	143	0	60	4	Na
Blizzard, Oreo cookies	Small	570	21	Na	12.5	<1	64	0	35	2	Na
Blizzard, Oreo cookies	Large	1010	37	Na	23	2	113	0	60	4	Na
Chocolate dilly bar	1	220	13	Na	11	2	20	0	10	0	Na
Classic banana split	1	510	12	Na	8	3	82	0	25	25	Na
DQ fudge bar	1	50	0	0	0	0	3	0	10	0	0
DQ vanilla orange bar	1	60	0	0	0	0	2	0	6	0	0
Peanut butter Blast	1	700	37	Na	19	2	64	0	25	2	Na

128

Food	Portion Size	Calories	Total Fat (g)	Good Fats (g)	Bad Fats (g)	Fiber (g)	Sugars (mg)	Beta-carotene (mcg)	Calcium (%DV)	Vit. C (%DV)	B vit. (0,+,++)
Starkiss bar	1	80	0	0	0	0	21	0	0	0	0
Sundae, chocolate	Small	280	7	Na	4.5	0	42	0	20	0	0
Sundae, strawberry	Large	500	15	Na	9	<1	72	0	40	30	0
Vanilla cone	Medium	330	9	Na	6	0	38	0	25	4	Na
Sandwiches, Sides											
Bacon cheddar grillburger	1	710	45	Na	23.5	1	8	0	25	4	Na
California grillburger	1	630	42	Na	16	1	5	0	10	8	Na
Classic grillburger, no cheese	1	540	30	Na	14	2	8	0	10	10	Na
Classic hot dog	1	240	14	Na	5	1	4	0	6	6	Na
Classic hot dog, chili cheese	1	330	21	Na	9	2	4	0	15	6	Na
Crispy chicken salad, no dressing or croutons	1	350	20	Na	8.5	6	9	Na	15	60	Na
Crispy chicken sandwich	1	590	34	Na	8	5	8	Na	15	4	Na
French fries	Regular	380	15	Na	7	<1	4	0	2	20	Na
French fries	Large	530	21	Na	10	<1	6	0	4	30	Na
Grilled chicken salad, no dressing	1	240	10	Na	5	4	7	Na	15	60	Na
Grilled chicken sandwich	1	340	16	Na	2.5	2	4	0	6	15	Na
Half lb grillburger, no cheese	1	800	50	Na	25.5	2	8	0	15	10	Na
Onion rings	4 oz	470	30	Na	13	3	7	0	4	30	Na
Onion rings	5 oz	590	37	Na	16	4	9	0	4	15	Na
FAST FOOD, Dunkin Donuts											
Bagels											
Cinnamon raisin	1	330	3	Na	0.5	3	11	0	4	0	+*
Everything	1	370	6	Na	0.5	3	4	0	6	0	+
Multigrain	1	380	6	Na	1	5	7	0	4	0	+

Food	Portion Size	Calories	Total Fat (g)	Good Fats (g)	Bad Fats (g)	Fiber (g)	Sugars (mg)	Beta-carotene (mcg)	Calcium (%DV)	Vit. C (%DV)	B vit. (0,+,++)
Plain	1	320	2.5	Na	0.5	2	4	0	0	0	+
Sesame	1	380	8	Na	0.5	3	4	0	0	0	+
Wheat	1	350	4	Na	1	4	7	0	0	0	+
Bakery											
Apple Danish	1	330	20	Na	9	1	10	0	0	0	+*
Biscuit	1	250	13	Na	11.5	1	3	0	4	0	Na
Blueberry muffin	1	470	17	Na	3	2	38	0	4	0	+*
Chocolate chip muffin	1	630	26	Na	8	2	49	0	4	0	+*
Coffee cake muffin	1	580	19	Na	3	1	40	0*	4	0	+*
Corn muffin	1	510	18	Na	3.5	1	32	33*	2	0	+*
Plain croissant	1	330	18	Na	11.5	0	3	25*	0	0	0
Beverages											
Caramel crème latte	10 oz	260	9	Na	6	0	40	0	30	0	0
Coffee Coolatta w/2% milk	16 oz	190	2	Na	1.5	0	40	0	15	0	0
Coffee Coolatta w/cream	16 oz	350	22	Na	14	0	35	0	10	0	0
Dunkaccino	10 oz	230	10	Na	8	0	25	0	4	0	0
Flavored coffees, all	10 oz	20	0	0	0	0	0	0	0	0	0
Iced coffee w/skim milk & sugar	16 oz	70	0	0	0	0	12	0	4	0	0
Cream Cheese											
Chive	2 oz	170	17	Na	11	2	2	50*	8	0	0
Garden vegetable	2 oz	170	15	Na	11	0	2	50*	4	0	0
Lite	2 oz	110	9	Na	7	0	3	25*	6	0	0
Salmon	2 oz	170	17	Na	11	0	0	50*	0	0	0
Strawberry	2 oz	190	17	Na	9	0	9	50*	4	4	0

Donuts and Fancies

Food	Portion Size	Calories	Total Fat (g)	Good Fats (g)	Bad Fats (g)	Fiber (g)	Sugars (mg)	Beta-carotene (mcg)	Calcium (%DV)	Vit. C (%DV)	B vit. (0,+,++)
Apple crumb	1	230	10	Na	3.5	1	12	0	0	0	0
Apple fritter	1	300	14	Na	5.5	1	12	0	0	0	0
Apple & spice	1	200	8	Na	4	1	7	0	0	0	0
Bavarian kreme	1	210	9	Na	4.5	1	9	0	0	0	0
Blueberry cake	1	290	16	Na	6	1	16	0	0	0	0
Boston kreme	1	240	9	Na	5.5	1	14	0	0	0	0
Chocolate frosted donut	1	200	9	Na	7	1	10	0	0	0	0
Chocolate glazed cake	1	290	16	Na	7.5	1	14	0	0	0	0
Chocolate iced bismark	1	340	15	Na	5	1	31	0	0	0	0
Chocolate kreme filled	1	270	13	Na	7	1	16	0	0	0	0
Cinnamon cake stick	1	450	30	Na	12	1	17	0	4	0	0
Cinnamon cake munchkins	4	270	15	Na	7.5	1	14	0	2	0	0
Éclair	1	270	11	Na	3	1	17	0	0	0	0
French cruller	1	150	8	Na	5	1	8	0	0	0	0
Glazed cake munchkins	3	280	13	Na	7	1	22	0	4	0	0
Glazed chocolate cake stick	1	470	29	Na	12	2	24	0	4	0	0
Glazed fritter	1	260	14	Na	5.5	1	7	0	0	0	0
Jelly filled munchkins	5	210	9	Na	4.5	1	15	0	0	0	0
Jelly filled stick	1	530	29	Na	12	1	32	0	2	0	0
Old fashioned cake donut	1	300	19	Na	9	1	9	0	2	0	0
Plain cake munchkins	4	270	16	Na	8	1	15	0	2	0	0
Plain cake stick	1	420	29	Na	12	1	12	0	2	0	0
Powdered cake donut	1	330	19	Na	9	1	17	0	2	0	0

Food	Portion Size	Calories	Total Fat (g)	Good Fats (g)	Bad Fats (g)	Fiber (g)	Sugars (mg)	Beta-carotene (mcg)	Calcium (%DV)	Vit. C (%DV)	B vit. (0,+,++)
Sugar raised donut	1	170	8	Na	2	1	4	0	0	0	0
Vanilla crème filled	1	270	13	Na	6.5	1	17	0	0	0	0
Sandwiches											
Bacon egg cheese croissant	1	520	33	Na	17	0	9	0	10	0	Na
Ham cheese bagel	1	510	16	Na	6	2	10	0	10	0	Na
Ham, egg, cheese croissant	1	520	32	Na	17	0	9	0	10	0	Na
Meatball Panini	1	480	19	Na	9	3	6	0	10	10	Na
Steak Panini	1	450	12	Na	5.5	3	4	0	20	0	Na
Southwestern chicken Panini	1	420	10	Na	5	3	4	0	15	4	Na
Supreme omelet croissant	1	590	38	Na	19	1	4	0	15	15	Na
FAST FOOD, KFC											
Sandwiches, Entrees											
Chicken pot pie	1	770	40	Na	29	5	2	Na	0	0	Na
KFC Snacker	1	320	16	Na	4.5	2	5	Na	6	4	Na
KFC Snacker sandwich, fish	1	280	7	Na	1.5	1	5	0	6	0	Na
KFC Snacker, ultimate cheese	1	280	11	Na	4.5	2	5	0	8	4	Na
Oven roasted chicken, drumstick	1	140	8	Na	3	0	0	0	2	0	Na
Oven roasted chicken, whole wing	1	150	9	Na	3.5	0	0	0	2	0	Na
Popcorn chicken, individual serving	1	370	24	Na	7	2	0	0	4	0	Na
Popcorn chicken	Large	560	31	Na	14	2	0	0	4	0	Na
Sides, Desserts											
Apple pie slice	1 slice	230	11	Na	4.5	2	23	0	2	0	Na
Baked Cheetos	1 serv	120	4.5	Na	1	0	1	0	0	0	0
Fiery buffalo wings	6	440	26	Na	10.5	2	1	0	4	35	Na

Food	Portion Size	Calories	Total Fat (g)	Good Fats (g)	Bad Fats (g)	Fiber (g)	Sugars (mg)	Beta-carotene (mcg)	Calcium (%DV)	Vit. C (%DV)	B vit. (0,+,++)
Hot wings	6	450	29	Na	10	2	0	0	4	2	Na
Lil Bucket chocolate cream	1	280	13	Na	10	3	21	0	4	0	Na
Lil Bucket strawberry shortcake	1	210	7	Na	5	3	21	0	4	0	Na
Mashed potatoes w/gravy	1 serv	140	5	Na	1.5	1	1	0	4	2	Na
Seasoned rice	1 serv	150	1	Na	0	1	1	0	4	0	Na
Sweet 'n spicy wings	6	460	26	Na	10.5	2	15	0	6	35	Na
FAST FOOD, McDonald's											
Beverages & Desserts											
Chocolate triple thick shake	16 oz	580	10	Na	6.5	1	84	Na	45	0	Na
Fruit yogurt parfait	1	160	2	Na	1	1	21	Na	15	15	Na
McDonaldland cookies	2 oz	250	8	Na	4.5	1	14	0	0	0	0
McFlurry w/MMs	1	620	20	Na	13	1	85	0	45	0	0
Orange juice	Small	140	0	0	0	0	29	Na	2	160	+
Vanilla triple thick shake	16 oz	550	13	Na	9	0	75	Na	45	0	Na
Breakfast											
Biscuit	Regular	230	10	Na	7	1	2	0	4	0	Na
Egg McMuffin	1	300	12	Na	4.5	2	3	0	30	0	Na
Hash browns	1 serv	140	8	Na	3.5	2	0	0	0	2	0
Hotcakes, margarine & syrup	1 serv	610	18	Na	8	3	47	0	15	0	Na
Sausage burrito	1	300	16	Na	7	1	2	0	15	0	Na
Sausage, egg, cheese McGriddle	1 serv	560	32	Na	12	2	15	0	20	0	Na
Sausage McMuffin w/egg	1	450	27	Na	10.5	2	2	0	30	0	Na
Sausage patty	1	170	15	Na	6	0	0	0	2	0	Na
Scrambled eggs (2)	1 serv	170	11	4.5*	4	0	0	30*	6	0	+

133

Food	Portion Size	Calories	Total Fat (g)	Good Fats (g)	Bad Fats (g)	Fiber (g)	Sugars (mg)	Beta-carotene (mcg)	Calcium (%DV)	Vit. C (%DV)	B vit. (0,+,++)
Sandwiches, Sides											
Bacon ranch salad grilled chicken	1	260	9	Na	4	3	5	0	15	50	Na
Big Mac	1	540	29	Na	11.5	3	9	0	25	2	Na
Big N Tasty	1	460	24	Na	9.5	3	8	0	15	8	Na
Caesar salad w/crispy chicken	1	300	13	Na	5.5	3	4	0	20	50	Na
Cheeseburger	1	300	12	Na	6.5	2	6	0	20	2	Na
Chicken Selects breast strips	3 pcs	380	20	Na	6	0	0	0	2	4	+
Chicken McNuggets	6 pcs	250	15	Na	4.5	0	0	0	2	2	+
Double cheeseburger	1	440	23	Na	12.5	2	7	0	25	2	Na
French fries	Small	250	13	Na	6	3	0	0	2	6	0
French fries	Large	570	30	Na	14	7	0	0	2	15	0
McChicken	1	360	16	Na	4.5	1	5	0	10	2	Na
Premium grilled chicken club sandwich	1	570	21	Na	7	4	12	0	20	10	Na
Quarterpounder w/cheese	1	510	25	Na	13.5	3	9	0	30	4	Na
FAST FOOD, Starbucks											
Caffe latte	16 oz	260	14	Na	9	0	19	0	0	0	0
Caffe vanilla frappuccino, no whip	16 oz	340	3.5	Na	2	0	63	0	0	0	0
Cappuccino	16 oz	150	8	Na	5	0	11	0	0	0	0
Caramel apple cider, no whip	16 oz	300	0	0	0	0	64	0	0	0	0
Iced caffe latte	16 oz	160	8	Na	5	0	11	0	0	0	0
Iced caffe mocha, whip	16 oz	350	20	Na	12.5	2	27	0	0	0	0
Iced tazo green tea latte	16 oz	250	8	Na	4.5	1	36	0	0	0	0
Tazo black tea lemonade	16 oz	120	0	0	0	0	29	0	0	0	0
Tazo chai tea latte	16 oz	290	7	Na	4.5	0	46	0	0	0	0

Food	Portion Size	Calories	Total Fat (g)	Good Fats (g)	Bad Fats (g)	Fiber (g)	Sugars (mg)	Beta-carotene (mcg)	Calcium (%DV)	Vit. C (%DV)	B vit. (0,+,++)
Toffee nut crème w/whip	16 oz	450	24	Na	15	0	42	0	0	0	0
Vanilla latte	16 oz	320	12	Na	7	0	36	0	0	0	0
FAST FOOD, Subway											
Breakfast Sandwiches and Wraps											
Cheese on Deli Round	1	310	12	Na	6	3	2	Na	15	6	Na
Cheese on 6-inch bread	1	350	12	Na	6	3	5	Na	20	15	Na
Chipotle steak & cheese on Deli Round	1	490	25	Na	9.5	4	5	Na	15	14	Na
Chipotle steak & cheese wrap	1	450	27	Na	8.5	9	3	Na	25	8	Na
Double bacon & cheese on Deli Round	1	410	19	Na	9.5	3	3	Na	15	6	Na
Double bacon & cheese wrap	1	360	21	Na	9	8	1	Na	25	0	Na
Honey mustard ham & egg on Deli Round	1	270	5	Na	1.5	3	9	Na	0	6	Na
Honey mustard ham & egg wrap	1	230	7	Na	1	8	6	Na	8	0	Na
Western w/cheese on Deli Round	1	350	13	Na	6	3	3	Na	15	8	Na
Western w/cheese wrap	1	300	15	Na	6	8	1	Na	25	8	Na
Western w/cheese on 6-inch bread	1	380	13	Na	6	4	6	Na	20	20	Na
6-Inch Sandwiches											
Chicken & Bacon Ranch	1	540	25	Na	10.5	5	7	Na	25	35	Na
Chicken parmesan	1	500	18	Na	6	5	8	Na	25	35	Na
Cold Cut Combo	1	410	17	Na	7.5	4	8	Na	15	35	Na
Ham	1	290	5	Na	1.5	4	8	Na	6	30	Na
Meatball marinara	1	560	24	Na	12	7	13	Na	20	60	Na
Roast beef	1	290	5	Na	2	4	8	Na	6	30	Na
Steak & cheese	1	400	12	Na	6.5	4	9	Na	15	50	Na
Subway melt	1	380	12	Na	5	4	8	Na	15	30	Na

Food	Portion Size	Calories	Total Fat (g)	Good Fats (g)	Bad Fats (g)	Fiber (g)	Sugars (mg)	Beta-carotene (mcg)	Calcium (%DV)	Vit. C (%DV)	B vit. (0,+,++)
Turkey breast	1	280	4.5	Na	1.5	4	7	Na	6	30	Na
Veggie Delite	1	230	3	Na	1	4	7	Na	6	30	Na
Deli Style & Wraps											
Chicken & bacon ranch w/cheese wrap	1	440	27	Na	10.5	9	1	Na	30	15	Na
Ham sandwich	1	210	4	Na	1.5	3	4	Na	8	20	Na
Roast beef sandwich	1	220	4.5	Na	2	3	4	Na	8	20	Na
Tuna w/cheese wrap	1	440	32	Na	6.5	9	1	Na	15	10	Na
Turkey breast & bacon w/chipotle, wrap	1	380	24	Na	7	9	2	Na	20	10	Na
Turkey breast wrap	1	190	6	Na	1	9	2	Na	10	10	Na
Double Meat 6-Inch Subs											
DM Chipotle southwest cheese steak	1	540	28	Na	11	5	8	Na	13	35	Na
DM cold cut combo	1	550	28	Na	11	4	8	Na	20	35	Na
DM ham	1	350	7	Na	2.5	4	9	Na	6	30	Na
DM Italian BMT	1	630	35	Na	14	4	10	Na	15	35	Na
DM meatball marinara	1	860	42	Na	20	10	18	Na	25	80	Na
DM oven roasted chicken	1	400	8	Na	2.5	5	11	Na	6	50	Na
DM roast beef	1	360	7	Na	3.5	4	9	Na	6	30	Na
DM subway club	1	420	8	Na	3.5	5	10	Na	8	30	Na
DM turkey breast	1	340	6	Na	1.5	4	8	Na	6	30	Na
DM turkey breast, ham & bacon melt	1	500	17	Na	8	4	9	Na	15	30	Na
Desserts											
Chocolate chip cookie	1	210	10	Na	6	1	18	0	0	0	0
Double chocolate chip cookie	1	210	10	Na	5	1	20	0	2	0	0
Oatmeal raisin cookie	1	200	8	Na	4	1	17	Na	2	0	Na

Food	Portion Size	Calories	Total Fat (g)	Good Fats (g)	Bad Fats (g)	Fiber (g)	Sugars (mg)	Beta-carotene (mcg)	Calcium (%DV)	Vit. C (%DV)	B vit. (0,+,++)
Peanut butter cookie	1	220	12	Na	5	1	16	Na	2	0	Na
Pie, apple	1	245	10	Na	2	1	25	Na	0	0	Na
White chip macadamia nut cookie	1	220	11	Na	5	<1	18	Na	2	0	Na
Salads											
Grilled chicken & baby spinach	1	140	3	Na	1	4	4	Na	10	80	Na
Subway club	1	160	4	Na	1.5	4	7	Na	6	50	Na
Tuna w/cheese	1	360	29	Na	6.5	4	5	Na	15	50	Na
Veggie Delite	1	60	1	0	0	4	5	Na	6	50	Na
Soups											
Brown & wild rice w/chicken	10 oz	220	11	Na	3.5	1	3	Na	15	50	Na
Chicken & dumpling	10 oz	140	3.5	Na	1.5	2	1	Na	4	0	Na
Chili con carne	10 oz	340	11	Na	5	10	7	Na	6	0	Na
Cream of broccoli	10 oz	140	5	Na	2	4	4	Na	15	20	Na
Cream of potato w/bacon	10 oz	220	10	Na	4	5	4	Na	10	0	Na
Minestrone	10 oz	90	0.5	0	0	4	4	Na	4	4	Na
New England clam chowder	10 oz	150	5	Na	1	2	2	Na	10	2	Na
Roasted chicken noodle	10 oz	90	1.5	Na	0.5	1	2	Na	2	2	Na
Spanish chicken w/rice	10 oz	110	2	Na	0.5	1	1	Na	2	4	Na
Tomato garden vegetable w/rotini	10 oz	100	1	0	0.5	3	8	Na	6	4	Na
FAST FOOD, Taco Bell											
Big Bell Value Menu											
Cheesy fiesta potatoes	1 serv	290	18	Na	9	2	2	Na	6	2	Na
Double decker taco	1	340	14	Na	6.5	5	2	Na	15	2	Na
Grande soft taco	1	450	21	Na	10.5	2	4	Na	20	2	Na

Food	Portion Size	Calories	Total Fat (g)	Good Fats (g)	Bad Fats (g)	Fiber (g)	Sugars (mg)	Beta-carotene (mcg)	Calcium (%DV)	Vit. C (%DV)	B vit. (0,+,++)
Spicy chicken soft taco	1	180	7	Na	2	2	2	Na	8	6	Na
Spicy chicken burrito	1	420	19	Na	5.5	4	4	Na	15	6	Na
½ lb beef combo burrito	1	470	19	Na	9	5	4	Na	20	8	Na
½ lb beef & potato burrito	1	540	25	Na	8	4	4	Na	20	8	Na
Burritos											
Bean	1	370	10	Na	5.5	8	4	Na	20	8	Na
Burrito supreme, beef	1	440	18	Na	10	5	5	Na	20	15	Na
Burrito supreme, chicken	1	410	14	Na	8	5	5	Na	20	15	Na
Burrito supreme, steak	1	420	16	Na	9	6	5	Na	20	15	Na
Fiesta burrito, beef	1	390	14	Na	7	3	4	Na	20	6	Na
Fiesta burrito, chicken	1	370	11	Na	5	3	4	Na	20	6	Na
Fiesta burrito, steak	1	370	12	Na	5.5	3	4	Na	20	4	Na
Grilled stuft burrito, beef	1	720	32	Na	14	7	6	Na	35	6	Na
Grilled stuft burrito, chicken	1	670	25	Na	9.5	7	6	Na	30	10	Na
Grilled stuft burrito, steak	1	690	27	Na	11	7	6	Na	30	6	Na
Chalupas											
Chalupa supreme, beef	1	400	24	Na	10.5	2	4	Na	15	6	Na
Chalupa supreme, chicken	1	370	21	Na	9	2	4	Na	15	8	Na
Chalupa supreme, steak	1	370	22	Na	9	2	4	Na	15	6	Na
Chalupa baja, beef	1	450	28	Na	9	2	4	Na	15	6	Na
Chalupa baja, chicken	1	400	24	Na	7	2	4	Na	15	6	Na
Chalupa baja, steak	1	410	25	Na	8	2	4	Na	15	6	Na
Chalupa nacho cheese, beef	1	380	22	Na	8	2	4	Na	10	8	Na

Food	Portion Size	Calories	Total Fat (g)	Good Fats (g)	Bad Fats (g)	Fiber (g)	Sugars (mg)	Beta-carotene (mcg)	Calcium (%DV)	Vit. C (%DV)	B vit. (0,+,++)
Chalupa nacho cheese, chicken	1	350	18	Na	7	2	4	Na	10	8	Na
Chalupa nacho cheese, steak	1	360	20	Na	7.5	2	4	Na	10	6	Na
Nachos & Sides											
Cinnamon twists	1	160	5	Na	2	<1	10	Na	0	0	0
Mexican rice	1 serv	200	9	Na	4	2	0	Na	10	0	Na
Nachos	1	320	20	Na	8.5	2	3	Na	8	0	Na
Nachos supreme	1	460	26	Na	11.5	5	3	Na	10	8	Na
Nachos BelGrande	1	790	44	Na	19	10	5	Na	15	10	Na
Tacos											
Crunchy taco	1	170	10	Na	4.5	<1	<1	Na	6	0	Na
Double decker taco supreme	1	360	18	Na	10	5	4	Na	15	6	Na
Grilled steak soft taco	1	280	17	Na	5.5	1	3	Na	10	6	Na
Ranchero chicken soft taco	1	270	14	Na	4.5	2	3	Na	10	8	Na
Soft taco, beef	1	210	10	Na	5	<1	2	Na	10	0	Na
Soft taco supreme, beef	1	260	14	Na	8	1	3	Na	15	6	Na
FAST FOOD, Wendy's											
Frosty											
Chocolate frosty, original, Jr.	1	160	4	Na	2.5	0	21	Na	15	0	Na
Chocolate frosty, original, small	1	330	8	Na	5	0	42	Na	30	0	Na
Chocolate frosty, original, medium	1	430	11	Na	7	0	55	Na	40	0	Na
Chocolate frosty, original, Fix 'N Mix	1	170	4	Na	2.5	0	22	Na	15	0	Na
Vanilla frosty, Jr.	1	150	4	Na	2.5	0	21	Na	15	0	Na
Vanilla frosty, small	1	310	8	Na	5	0	43	Na	30	0	Na

Food	Portion Size	Calories	Total Fat (g)	Good Fats (g)	Bad Fats (g)	Fiber (g)	Sugars (mg)	Beta-carotene (mcg)	Calcium (%DV)	Vit. C (%DV)	B vit. (B,+,++)
Vanilla frosty, medium	1	410	10	Na	6	0	57	Na	40	0	Na
Vanilla frosty, Fix 'N Mix	1	160	4	Na	2.5	0	22	Na	15	0	Na
Salads											
Caesar chicken salad	1	190	5	Na	2.5	4	4	Na	20	90	Na
Chicken BLT salad	1	340	18	Na	9	4	6	Na	30	50	Na
Mandarin chicken salad	1	170	2	Na	0.5	3	13	Na	6	50	Na
Southwest taco salad	1	440	22	Na	13	9	10	Na	45	35	Na
Sandwiches											
Big bacon classic	1	590	30	Na	13.5	3	11	Na	15	15	Na
Black forest ham & swiss Frescata	1	470	19	Na	6	4	8	Na	20	20	Na
Cheeseburger, kids' meal	1	320	13	Na	6.5	1	7	Na	10	0	Na
Chicken club sandwich	1	650	31	Na	11.5	2	8	Na	40	8	Na
Classic single w/everything	1	420	20	Na	8	2	8	Na	4	8	Na
Crispy chicken sandwich	1	380	14	Na	2.5	1	5	Na	2	2	Na
Deluxe crispy chicken sandwich	1	450	19	Na	5	2	7	Na	10	8	Na
Double Jr cheeseburger deluxe	1	460	23	Na	10	2	8	Na	10	8	Na
Frescata club	1	440	17	Na	3.5	4	5	Na	2	15	Na
Ham & cheese sandwich, kids' meal	1	240	6	Na	3	1	6	Na	8	2	Na
Homestyle chicken fillet sandwich	1	470	16	Na	3	2	8	Na	4	8	Na
Jr. bacon cheeseburger	1	370	17	Na	7.5	2	6	Na	10	6	Na
Jr. cheeseburger deluxe	1	360	16	Na	6.5	2	8	Na	10	6	Na
Jr. cheeseburger	1	280	9	Na	4	1	7	Na	2	0	Na
Roasted turkey & basil pesto Frescata	1	420	15	Na	3	4	3	Na	6	35	Na
Roasted turkey & swiss Frescata	1	480	20	Na	6	4	4	Na	20	15	Na

Food	Portion Size	Calories	Total Fat (g)	Good Fats (g)	Bad Fats (g)	Fiber (g)	Sugars (mg)	Beta-carotene (mcg)	Calcium (%DV)	Vit. C (%DV)	B vit. (0,+,++)
Spicy chicken fillet sandwich	1	480	17	Na	3	4	8	Na	4	8	Na
Ultimate chicken grill sandwich	1	370	8	Na	1.5	2	10	Na	4	10	Na
Sides and Nuggets											
Caesar side salad w/o dressing	1	80	4.5	Na	2	2	1	Na	10	35	Na
Chili	Small	220	6	Na	2.5	5	6	Na	8	4	Na
Chili	Large	330	9	Na	4	8	9	Na	10	6	Na
French fries	Small	370	18	Na	3.5	5	0	Na	2	8	Na
French fries	Large	540	26	Na	5	7	0	Na	2	10	Na
Nuggets, 4 piece kids' meal	4 pcs	190	12	Na	2	0	1	Na	2	0	Na
Nuggets, 10 piece	10 pcs	460	30	Na	6	0	1	Na	2	0	Na
Sour cream & chives baked potato	1	320	4	Na	2.5	7	4	Na	8	60	Na
FIGS											
Canned, solids & liquid	1 c	131	0	0	0	5	29	57	7	4	0
Fresh, large 2.5"	1	47	0	0	0	2	10	54	2	2	0
Stewed	1 c	277	1	0	0	11	60	7	18	19	+
SunMaid, mission & calimyrna	4	120	0	0	0	5	21	Na	6	3	0
FILBERTS, dry roasted, no salt	1 oz	182	18	13	2	3	1	10	3	1	0
FLOUNDER, baked	3 oz	99	1	0	0	0	0	0	1	0	+
FLOUR											
Barley	1 c	511	2	Na	0	15	1	0	4	0	+
Corn, whole grain, yellow	1 c	422	5	1	1	16	1	113	0	0	+
Cornmeal, self-rising, enriched	1 c	489	2	0.5	0	10	1	0	48	0	‡
Gold Medal, unbleached, all-purpose	¼ c	100	0	0	0	1	1	Na	0	0	Na

Food	Portion Size	Calories	Total Fat (g)	Good Fats (g)	Bad Fats (g)	Fiber (g)	Sugars (mg)	Beta-carotene (mcg)	Calcium (%DV)	Vit. C (%DV)	B vit. (0,+,++)
Rice, brown	1 c	574	4.5	1.5	1	7	0	0	2	0	+
Rye, dark	1 c	415	3	0.5	0	29	1	0	7	0	Na
FRANKFURTERS											
Ballpark											
Beef franks	1	180	16	Na	7	0	2	0	0	6	0
Bun size smoked white turkey	1	45	0	0	0	0	3	0	0	6	0
Grillmaster deli style	1	250	23	Na	9	0	1	0	0	12	0
Grillmaster hearty beef	1	250	23	Na	9	0	1	0	0	8	0
Hebrew National											
97% fat free beef	1	45	1.5	Na	1	0	0	0	0	0	0
1/4 lb dinner frank	1	350	32	Na	15	0	0	0	0	0	0
Beef frank	1	150	14	Na	6	0	0	0	0	0	0
Cocktail franks	5 links	180	16	Na	7	0	0	0	0	0	0
Oscar Mayer											
Beef bun-length	1	180	17	Na	8	0	0	0	6	0	0
Beef franks	1	140	13	Na	7	0	1	0	0	0	0
Beef jumbo	1	180	17	Na	8	0	1	0	6	0	0
Cheese dogs	1	140	13	Na	4	0	0	0	6	0	0
Turkey franks	1	100	8	Na	2.5	0	1	0	2	0	0
FRANKFURTER SUBSTITUTES											
Morningstar veggie dog	1	80	0.5	0	0	2	2	0	0	0	+
Morningstar corn dog	1	150	4	1	0.5	3	4	0	0	0	Na
Worthington big franks	1	118	7	1.5	0.5	1.5	0	Na	1	0	+
Yves, hot & spicy chili veggie	1	74	1	0	0	2	1	Na	2	0	+

Food	Portion Size	Calories	Total Fat (g)	Good Fats (g)	Bad Fats (g)	Fiber (g)	Sugars (mg)	Beta-carotene (mcg)	Calcium (%DV)	Vit. C (%DV)	B vit. (0,+,++)
Yves, tofu dog	1	47	0.5	0	0	0	0	Na	2	0	0
Yves, veggie dog	1	56	0	0	0	1	0	Na	2	0	+
FRENCH TOAST											
Aunt Jemima cinnamon French toast	2 slices	240	7	Na	1.5	2	6	0	10	0	0
Dunkables French toast sticks	6 sticks	240	7	Na	3.5	2	11	Na	8	0	+
FROSTING											
Betty Crocker											
Rich & Creamy butter cream	2 tbs	140	5	Na	3	0	20	0	0	0	0
Rich & Creamy caramel	2 tbs	140	5	Na	3	0	20	0	0	0	0
Rich & Creamy cherry	2 tbs	150	7	Na	4.5	0	20	0	0	0	0
Rich & Creamy coconut pecan	2 tbs	140	7	Na	4.5	<1	16	0	0	0	0
Rich & Creamy vanilla	2 tbs	140	5	Na	3	0	20	0	0	0	0
Whipped butter cream	2 tbs	110	5	Na	3	0	13	0	0	0	0
Whipped chocolate	2 tbs	100	5	Na	2.5	1	12	0	0	0	0
Whipped cream cheese	2 tbs	110	5	Na	3	0	13	0	0	0	0
Whipped milk chocolate	2 tbs	100	4.5	Na	2.5	0	12	0	0	0	0
Whipped vanilla	2 tbs	110	5	Na	3	0	13	0	0	0	0
Whipped whipped cream	2 tbs	100	5	Na	3	0	13	0	0	0	0
FROZEN BREAKFAST											
Amy's Kitchen, breakfast burrito	1	250	7	Na	0.5	5	4	Na	6	10	Na
Jimmy Dean wrap, sausage, egg, cheese	1	320	17	0.5	7.5	5	5	0	30	0	++
Pillsbury Toaster Scramble bacon & sausage	1	180	12	Na	5	0	1	Na	0	0	Na
Pillsbury Toaster Scramble cheese, egg, bacon	1	180	12	Na	5	0	1	Na	0	0	Na
South Beach Diet breakfast wrap, all-American	1	230	9	Na	3	6	3	Na	25	0	Na

Food	Portion Size	Calories	Total Fat (g)	Good Fats (g)	Bad Fats (g)	Fiber (g)	Sugars (mg)	Beta-carotene (mcg)	Calcium (%DV)	Vit. C (%DV)	B vit. (0,+,++)
South Beach Diet breakfast wrap, Denver	1	210	8	Na	2.5	6	3	Na	20	4	Na
South Beach Diet breakfast wrap, SW style	1	190	6	Na	2	6	2	Na	15	6	Na
South Beach Diet breakfast wrap, vegetable	1	160	6	Na	3	15	2	Na	25	4	Na
FROZEN DINNERS & ENTREES											
Amy's Kitchen											
Asian noodle stir-fry	1 pkg	290	7	Na	1	4	16	0	10	50	Na
Black bean vegetable enchilada	1	180	6	Na	0.5	3	2	Na	4	10	Na
Broccoli pot pie	1	430	22	Na	10	4	3	Na	15	45	Na
Brown rice & vegetables bowl	1	260	9	Na	1	5	7	Na	8	35	Na
Country vegetable pie	1	370	16	Na	9	4	5	Na	20	30	Na
Indian matter paneer	1 pkg	320	8	Na	1.5	6	8	Na	10	30	Na
Indian samosa wraps	1 wrap	260	8	Na	1	4	3	Na	4	25	Na
Macaroni & cheese	9 oz pkg	410	16	Na	10	3	6	Na	30	2	Na
Mexican casserole bowl	1	470	16	Na	5	7	3	Na	25	6	Na
Non-dairy vegetable pot pie	1	360	13	Na	1.5	4	3	Na	6	15	Na
Pesto tortelli bowl	1	430	19	Na	8	3	5	Na	40	8	Na
Ravioli bowl	1	380	12	Na	4.5	4	7	Na	20	20	Na
Santa Fe enchilada bowl	1	350	11	Na	2	10	5	Na	10	40	Na
Shepherd's pie	1	160	4	Na	0	5	5	Na	10	30	Na
Stuffed pasta shells bowl	1	310	13	Na	7	5	7	Na	40	40	Na
Thai noodle stir-fry	1 pkg	310	11	Na	7	5	2	0	4	45	Na

Food	Portion Size	Calories	Total Fat (g)	Good Fats (g)	Bad Fats (g)	Fiber (g)	Sugars (mg)	Beta-carotene (mcg)	Calcium (%DV)	Vit. C (%DV)	B vit. (0,+,++)
Vegetable pot pie	1 meal	420	19	Na	12	4	3	Na	4	10	Na
Whole Meals: black bean enchilada	1 meal	330	8	Na	4	9	4	Na	6	20	Na
Whole Meals: cheese enchilada	1 meal	350	15	Na	7	6	6	Na	30	35	Na
Whole Meals: chili & cornbread	1 meal	340	6	Na	2.5	10	14	Na	10	25	Na
Whole Meals: veggie loaf	1 meal	280	7	Na	1	7	6	Na	4	50	Na
Birds Eye											
Alfredo chicken, cooked	1 c	320	17	Na	10	2	5	Na	10	20	Na
Beef steak & garlic potatoes, cooked	1 c	190	7	Na	2	3	4	Na	4	4	Na
Chicken fajita, cooked	1 c	150	6	Na	2	3	7	Na	2	70	Na
Garden herb chicken, cooked	1 c	280	11	Na	6	3	9	Na	10	10	Na
Garlic shrimp, cooked	1 c	220	8	Na	3.5	2	6	Na	6	25	Na
Pesto chicken primavera, cooked	1 c	210	7	Na	2	2	7	Na	10	30	Na
Teriyaki chicken, cooked	1 c	250	2.5	Na	0	2	12	Na	4	25	Na
Gorton's											
Beer batter fillets	2 fillets	230	14	Na	2.5	0	3	0	2	0	+
Classic grilled salmon	1 fillet	100	3.5	1.5	0.5	0	1	0	0	0	+
Crispy battered fillets	2 fillets	260	17	Na	3	0	3	0	2	0	+
Crunchy golden fillets	2 fillets	240	12	Na	2.5	0	3	0	2	0	+
Fish sticks	6 sticks	250	14	Na	3.5	0	2	0	2	0	+
Fried rice shrimp bowl	1	350	2.5	Na	0.5	1	9	0	10	4	+
Garlic & herb fish fillets	2 fillets	230	12	Na	2	0	4	0	2	0	+
Grilled fillets, Cajun blackened	1 fillet	100	3	Na	0.5	0	0	0	2	0	+
Grilled fillets, lemon pepper	1 fillet	100	3	Na	0.5	0	0	0	2	0	+
Original batter tenders	4 oz	270	15	Na	3	0	2	0	0	0	+

Food	Portion Size	Calories	Total Fat (g)	Good Fats (g)	Bad Fats (g)	Fiber (g)	Sugars (mg)	Beta-carotene (mcg)	Calcium (%DV)	Vit. C (%DV)	B vit. (0,+,++)
Parmesan breaded fillets	2 fillets	250	15	Na	3	0	5	0	2	0	+
Popcorn fish	11 pcs	280	17	Na	4.5	0	3	0	2	0	+
Popcorn shrimp, beer batter	18 pcs	270	16	Na	4.5	0	2	0	2	0	Na
Popcorn shrimp, original	20 pcs	240	12	Na	3.5	0	2	0	2	0	Na
Ranch fillets	2 fillets	240	13	Na	2.5	0	3	0	2	0	+
Teriyaki shrimp bowl	1	320	6	Na	1	2	14	0	15	40	Na
Green Giant—Complete Skillet Meals											
Chicken alfredo, prep.	1¼ c	270	4.5	Na	3	3	5	Na	10	25	Na
Chicken low mein, prep.	1 c	190	2	Na	0	3	7	0	4	40	0
Chicken teriyaki, prep.	1½ c	240	1	0	0	3	8	0	4	50	0
Garlic chicken pasta, prep.	1 c	230	6	Na	2.5	4	5	Na	6	25	0
Green Giant—Create A Meal											
Spicy Teriyaki, prep.	1 c	210	7	Na	1	3	9	0	4	70	Na
Stir-fry lo mein, prep.	1 c	270	7	Na	1.5	2	7	0	4	30	Na
Stir-fry sesame, prep.	1 c	260	12	Na	2	4	4	0	6	80	Na
Szechuan, prep.	1 c	190	9	Na	2.5	3	4	0	4	50	Na
Teriyaki, prep.	1 c	180	6	Na	1	3	3	Na	4	70	Na
Healthy Choice—Complete Selections											
Asiago chicken portabello	1 pkg	330	5	Na	2	7	12	0	8	8	0
Beef pot roast	1 pkg	310	Na	Na	3	5	21	0	4	30	0
Charbroiled beef patty	1 pkg	310	9	Na	3	6	9	0	4	6	0
Chicken enchilada suprema	1 pkg	352	8	2	3	5	2	0	5	0	0
Chicken mesquite BBQ	1 pkg	277	4	2	1	7	14	0	3	0	0
Chicken teriyaki w/rice	1 pkg	250	5	2	1.5	9	14	0	3	0	0

Food	Portion Size	Calories	Total Fat (g)	Good Fats (g)	Bad Fats (g)	Fiber (g)	Sugars (mg)	Beta-carotene (mcg)	Calcium (%DV)	Vit. C (%DV)	B vit. (0,+,++)
Country breaded chicken	1 pkg	370	9	Na	2	6	19	0	4	4	0
Creamy garlic shrimp	1 pkg	280	5	Na	1.5	5	16	0	10	8	0
Grilled turkey breast	1 pkg	270	3	0	1	5	26	0	8	80	0
Honey glazed chicken	1 pkg	270	6	Na	1.5	7	16	0	4	10	0
Lemon pepper fish	1 pkg	310	4.5	Na	1	5	14	0	2	50	0
Oven roasted beef	1 pkg	280	7	Na	2.5	5	7	0	2	10	0
Sesame chicken	1 pkg	330	8	Na	2	5	16	0	6	25	0
Sweet & sour chicken	1 pkg	430	9	Na	1	5	29	0	4	50	0
Traditional turkey breast	1 pkg	300	4	Na	1	6	20	0	4	10	0
Healthy Choice–Simple Selections											
Beef teriyaki	1 pkg	310	7	Na	2.5	5	17	0	2	4	0
Cheesy rice & chicken	1 pkg	220	6	Na	2.5	5	2	0	10	15	0
Chicken breast & vegetables	1 pkg	270	7	Na	2	56	4	0	4	10	0
Chicken fettuccini alfredo	1 pkg	210	5	Na	2	5	3	0	10	6	0
Chicken piccata	1 pkg	270	6	Na	2.5	2	5	0	2	10	0
Grilled chicken & mashed potatoes	1 pkg	160	3.5	Na	1.5	3	3	0	4	2	0
Lasagna bake	1 pkg	240	4.5	Na	1.5	5	10	0	10	6	0
Macaroni & cheese	1 pkg	210	5	Na	2	4	4	0	15	8	0
Oriental style chicken	1 pkg	230	4	Na	1	4	5	0	2	6	0
Sirloin beef tips & mushroom sauce	1 pkg	270	6	Na	2	4	2	0	2	0	0
Spaghetti w/meat sauce	1 pkg	220	3.5	Na	1	5	7	0	6	8	0
Lean Cuisine–Café Classics											
Beef Portobello	1 pkg	210	5	1.5	2.5	2	6	0	6	0	0
Chicken w/almonds	1 pkg	260	4.5	2	0.5	3	12	0	4	8	0

Food	Portion Size	Calories	Total Fat (g)	Good Fats (g)	Bad Fats (g)	Fiber (g)	Sugars (mg)	Beta-carotene (mcg)	Calcium (%DV)	Vit. C (%DV)	B vit. (0,+,++)
Chicken carbonara	1 pkg	270	6	2	2	2	5	0	10	10	0
Fiesta grilled chicken	1 pkg	250	7	2	3	3	8	0	15	40	0
Sweet & sour chicken	1 pkg	300	3	1	0.5	1	21	0	2	30	0
Three cheese chicken	1 pkg	220	9	2.5	3	2	5	0	15	40	0
Lean Cuisine—Comfort Classics											
Baked chicken	1 pkg	240	4.5	1	1	3	5	0	4	6	0
Baked lemon pepper fish	1 pkg	230	6	1.5	2	2	6	0	20	30	0
Beef pot roast	1 pkg	190	6	2.5	1.5	3	4	0	6	2	0
Beef peppercorn	1 pkg	220	7	2	2.5	3	8	0	10	20	0
Honey roasted pork	1 pkg	230	9	2.5	3.5	5	8	0	6	6	0
Roast turkey & vegetables	1 pkg	150	5	2	1	3	4	0	6	10	0
Southern beef tips	1 pkg	250	5	2	2	3	11	0	4	8	0
Lean Cuisine—Dinnertime Selects											
Chicken Florentine	1 pkg	390	8	2	3.5	6	13	0	35	0	0
Jumbo rigatoni w/meatballs	1 pkg	390	8	3	2.5	7	11	0	15	10	0
Orange peel chicken	1 pkg	390	9	3.5	1.5	3	15	0	8	25	0
Lean Cuisine—One Dish Favorites											
Cheese ravioli	1 pkg	250	6	1	3.5	3	10	0	15	2	0
Chicken chow mein w/rice	1 pkg	190	2.5	1	0.5	2	4	0	4	4	0
Chicken enchilada suiza	1 pkg	270	4.5	1	2	3	6.5	0	16	0	+
Four cheese cannelloni	1 pkg	240	7	2	3.5	3	9	0	25	4	0
Macaroni & beef	1 pkg	250	4.5	2	2	5	11	0	9	0	0
Spaghetti w/meat sauce	1 pkg	280	3.5	1.5	1.5	4.5	8	0	10	4	+
Spaghetti w/meatballs	1 pkg	250	5	2	2	4	6.5	0	10	0	+

Food	Portion Size	Calories	Total Fat (g)	Good Fats (g)	Bad Fats (g)	Fiber (g)	Sugars (mg)	Beta-carotene (mcg)	Calcium (%DV)	Vit. C (%DV)	B vit. (0,+,++)
Lean Cuisine—Skillets											
Asian style chicken & vegetables	1 pkg	160	2.5	0.5	0.5	2	5	0	2	4	0
Chicken alfredo	1 pkg	190	4.5	1	2	3	5	0	10	30	0
Chicken teriyaki	1 pkg	230	2	0.5	1	4	11	0	4	15	0
Three cheese chicken	1 pkg	200	5	1	2	3	5	0	15	20	0
Lean Cuisine—Spa Cuisine											
Chicken Mediterranean	1 pkg	220	4	1.5	0.5	3	6	0	10	4	0
Chicken in peanut sauce	1 pkg	280	8	3	1.5	3	6	0	10	8	0
Oven roasted beef burgundy	1 pkg	300	7	2	3	3	5	0	10	10	0
Pork w/cherry sauce	1 pkg	260	4	1.5	1.5	4	13	0	4	10	0
Rosemary chicken	1 pkg	220	4	1	2	3	1	0	6	10	0
Salmon w/basil	1 pkg	230	6	2	2	5	3	0	15	4	0
Stouffers—Entrees & Grilled Entrees											
Creamed chipped beef	1 pkg	138	7	2	4.5	0.5	4	0	10	0	+
Stuffed peppers w/beef	1 pkg	161	5.5	2	2.5	2.5	6	0	4	0	+
Weight Watchers—Smart Ones											
Angel hair marinara	1 pkg	230	1.5	Na	0.5	2	8	Na	2	6	Na
Broccoli & cheddar roasted potatoes	1 pkg	220	6	Na	3	5	3	Na	15	80	Na
Chicken carbonara	1 pkg	250	4.5	Na	1.5	2	<1	Na	10	2	Na
Chicken fettuccini	1 pkg	340	8	Na	4	4	2	Na	20	0	Na
Chicken Mirabella	1 pkg	180	2	Na	0.5	3	4	Na	6	15	Na
Chicken parmesan	1 pkg	290	5	Na	1.5	4	5	Na	20	10	Na
Creamy rigatoni w/broccoli & chicken	1 pkg	290	8	Na	3	2	4	Na	20	10	Na
Dragon shrimp lo mein	1 pkg	240	4	Na	1	3	5	Na	4	6	Na

149

Food	Portion Size	Calories	Total Fat (g)	Good Fats (g)	Bad Fats (g)	Fiber (g)	Sugars (mg)	Beta-carotene (mcg)	Calcium (%DV)	Vit. C (%DV)	B vit. (o,+,++)
Fajita chicken supreme	1 pkg	260	7	Na	3	4	3	Na	10	25	Na
Honey Dijon chicken	1 pkg	220	3.5	Na	0.5	2	8	Na	4	8	Na
Lasagna Florentine	1 pkg	290	9	Na	5	4	10	Na	30	4	Na
Meatloaf w/gravy	1 pkg	260	8	Na	2.5	5	1	Na	10	0	Na
Penne pollo	1 pkg	280	6	Na	2.5	3	5	0	15	20	0
Peppersteak	1 pkg	250	4.5	Na	1.5	3	4	Na	2	30	Na
Ravioli Florentine	1 pkg	250	5	Na	2	4	12	Na	15	15	Na
Roast beef w/gravy	1 pkg	210	9	Na	3	2	1	Na	2	8	Na
Salisbury steak	1 pkg	260	7	Na	3	3	2	Na	10	4	Na
Santa Fe style rice & beans	1 pkg	310	7	Na	3	4	6	Na	20	8	Na
Shrimp marinara	1 pkg	180	1.5	Na	0	4	4	Na	8	4	Na
Slow roasted turkey breast	1 pkg	210	7	Na	2	2	4	Na	2	6	Na
Southwest style adobe chicken	1 pkg	310	10	Na	3	3	5	Na	4	6	Na
Swedish meatballs	1 pkg	270	5	Na	2	3	4	Na	15	0	Na
Thai chicken & rice noodles	1 pkg	260	4	Na	0.5	2	9	Na	4	2	Na
Three cheese ziti marinara	1 pkg	290	7	Na	2.5	4	2	Na	15	2	Na
Tuna noodle gratin	1 pkg	250	4.5	Na	1.5	2	5	Na	15	0	Na
FROZEN SANDWICHES/POCKETS											
Amy's Kitchen											
Broccoli & cheese in a pocket sandwich	1	270	10	Na	4	3	4	Na	20	20	0
Cheese pizza in a pocket sandwich	1	300	9	Na	3.5	4	5	Na	20	6	0
Roasted vegetable in a pocket sandwich	1	230	8	Na	1.5	4	5	Na	2	10	0
Soy cheese pizza in a pocket sandwich	1	260	8	Na	0.5	1	3	Na	2	10	0
Spinach pizza in a pocket sandwich	1	280	9	Na	4	3	3	Na	20	10	0

Food	Portion Size	Calories	Total Fat (g)	Good Fats (g)	Bad Fats (g)	Fiber (g)	Sugars (mg)	Beta-carotene (mcg)	Calcium (%DV)	Vit. C (%DV)	B vit. (0,+,++)
Tofu scramble in a pocket sandwich	1	180	6	Na	0	<1	2	Na	0	20	0
Vegetable pie in a pocket sandwich	1	300	9	Na	1.5	3	5	Na	2	8	0
Croissant Pockets											
Ham & cheese	1	340	16	Na	8	2	14	Na	20	0	Na
Pepperoni pizza	1	390	20	Na	10	3	8	Na	20	0	+
Philly cheese steak	1	340	19	Na	8	3	6	Na	25	2	Na
Hot Pockets											
3 cheese & chicken quesadilla	1 pc	320	13	Na	6	3	7	Na	20	0	+
4 meat & 4 cheese	1 pc	300	19	Na	9	9	8	Na	20	0	+
Beef taco	1 pc	320	13	Na	6	5	5	Na	20	0	+
Chicken fajita	1 pc	290	11	Na	4	3	9	Na	15	0	+
Ham & cheese	1 pc	310	13	Na	5	3	7	Na	15	0	+
Meatballs & mozzarella	1 pc	330	14	Na	5	3	11	Na	20	0	+
Pepperoni pizza	1 pc	360	17	Na	6	3	12	Na	20	0	+
Supreme pizza	1 pc	350	15	Na	6	3	12	Na	20	0	+
Lean Pockets											
Cheeseburger	1 pc	280	7	Na	4	3	9	Na	25	0	Na
Chicken parmesan	1 pc	280	7	Na	3	3	5	Na	15	0	+
Philly steak & cheese	1 pc	280	7	Na	3.5	3	6	Na	20	0	+
Sausage, egg & cheese	1 pc	140	4.5	Na	1.5	2	4	Na	8	0	+
FRUIT SNACKS											
Betty Crocker Fruit by the Foot, all flavors	1 roll	80	1	0	0	0	10	0	0	25	0
Betty Crocker Fruit Roll Ups, all flavors	1 roll	50	1	0	0	0	7	0	0	25	0
Betty Crocker Fruit Flavored Shapes	1 pouch	80	0	0	0	0	14	0	0	100	0

Food	Portion Size	Calories	Total Fat (g)	Good Fats (g)	Bad Fats (g)	Fiber (g)	Sugars (mg)	Beta-carotene (mcg)	Calcium (%DV)	Vit. C (%DV)	B vit. (0,+,++)
GARLIC, raw	3 cloves	13	0	0	0	0	0	0	1	4	0
GELATIN											
Jell-O, all flavors, regular	½ c	80	0	0	0	0	0	0	0	0	0
Jell-O all flavors, sugar free	½ c	10	0	0	0	0	0	0	0	0	0
Royal, all flavors, regular	½ c	70	0	0	0	0	0	0	0	0	0
Royal, all flavors, sugar free	½ c	5	0	0	0	0	0	0	0	0	0
GRAPES, red or green	1 c	110	0	0	0	1	25	62	1	28	0
GRAPE JUICE/DRINK											
Capri Sun, Grape Tide	8 oz	100	0	0	0	0	23	0	0	0	0
Cascadian Farms, organic juice	8 oz	150	0	0	0	0	37	12*	0	0	0
Knudsen, 100% juice	8 oz	150	0	0	0	0	37	Na	2	4	0
Knudsen, concord grape	8 oz	160	0	0	0	0	39	Na	2	8	0
Kool-Aid, sugar-sweetened	8 oz	60	0	0	0	0	16	0	0	10	0
GRAPEFRUIT											
Fresh, pink or red, sections w/juice	1 c	96	0	0	0	4	16	1577	5	119	0
Fresh, white, sections w/juice	1 c	75	0	0	0	3	17	32	2	127	0
Del Monte, sections, red	½ c	90	0	0	0	1	17	780*	2	100	0
Del Monte, sun fresh red	½ c	80	0	0	0	2	9	780*	2	100	0
Del Monte, sun fresh white in real juice	½ c	45	0	0	0	2	8	16*	2	100	0
Fruit Naturals, red	½ c	60	0	0	0	<1	13	780*	2	100	0
GRAPEFRUIT JUICE											
Knudsen, organic	8 oz	100	0	0	0	0	23	Na	2	70	0
Minute Maid, 100% juice, frozen w/calcium	8 oz	100	0	0	0	0	20	0	10	140	0

Food	Portion Size	Calories	Total Fat (g)	Good Fats (g)	Bad Fats (g)	Fiber (g)	Sugars (mg)	Beta-carotene (mcg)	Calcium (%DV)	Vit. C (%DV)	B vit. (0,+,++)
Tropicana, 100% juice, ruby red	8 oz	90	0	0	0	0	17	Na	2	120	0
Tropicana, sweet grapefruit	8 oz	130	0	0	0	0	27	Na	2	100	+
GRAVY											
Boston Market, pan style poultry	2 oz	40	2	Na	1	0	0	0	0	0	0
Campbell's											
Beef	1/4 c	40	1	Na	0.5	0	<1	0	0	0	0
Chicken	1/4 c	40	3	Na	1	0	1	0	0	0	0
Country style cream	1/4 c	45	3	Na	1	0	1	0	0	0	0
Fat free chicken	1/4 c	15	0	0	0	0	0	0	0	0	0
Franco-American, beef, slow roast	1/4 c	25	1	Na	0.5	0	0	0	0	0	0
Franco-American, turkey, slow roast	1/4 c	25	1	Na	0.5	0	0	0	0	0	0
Franco-American, fat-free slow roast beef	1/4 c	20	1	Na	0.5	0	0	0	0	0	0
GREEN BEANS											
Fresh, boiled, no salt	1 c	44	0	0	0	4	2	417	4	29	0
Canned											
Del Monte, cut	1/2 c	20	0	0	0	2	2	0	2	4	0
Del Monte, cut Italian	1/2 c	30	0	0	0	3	2	0	2	4	0
Del Monte, cut w/potatoes and ham style	1/2 c	30	0	0	0	<1	1	0	2	8	0
Del Monte, French style	1/2 c	20	0	0	0	2	2	175*	2	4	0
Del Monte, seasoned	1/2 c	20	0	0	0	2	2	175*	2	4	0
S&W, cut	1/2 c	20	0	0	0	2	2	175*	2	4	0
Frozen											
Cascadian Farms, cut, organic	3/4 c	30	0	0	0	2	2	400*	2	8	0
Cascadian Farms, French w/almonds	2/3 c	70	3	Na	0	4	4	400*	6	20	0

Food	Portion Size	Calories	Total Fat (g)	Good Fats (g)	Bad Fats (g)	Fiber (g)	Sugars (mg)	Beta-carotene (mcg)	Calcium (%DV)	Vit. C (%DV)	B vit. (0,+,++)
Green Giant, cut	½ c	25	0	0	0	2	2	225*	4	6	0
Green Giant, casserole	⅔ c	110	8	Na	3.5	1	2	Na	2	6	0
HADDOCK, baked	3 oz	95	1	0	0	0	0	0	3	0	+
HALIBUT, Atlantic & Pacific, baked	3 oz	119	2	1	0	0	0	0	5	0	+
Greenland, baked	3 oz	203	15	9	3	0	0	0	0	0	+
HAM											
Cured, regular	3 oz	151	8	4	3	0	0	0	0	0	+
Fresh, leg, shank, lean & fat, roasted	3 oz	246	17	Na	6	0	0	0	1	0	+
Fresh, rump, lean & fat, roasted	3 oz	214	12	Na	4	0	0	0	1	0	+
Oscar Mayer, deli style, honey shaved	⅕ pkg	50	1	0	0.5	0	0	0	0	0	0
Oscar Mayer, smoked shaved	⅕ pkg	45	1	0	0	0	0	0	0	0	0
HAMBURGER MIX (mix only—unprep.)											
Beef pasta	⅓ c	110	1	Na	0	1	1	Na	0	0	+
Beef taco	½ c	140	1.5	Na	0	1	3	0	2	0	+
Cheeseburger macaroni	⅓ c	160	2.5	Na	1	0	3	0	0	0	0
Cheesy enchilada	⅓ c	170	1.5	Na	0.5	<1	3	0	6	0	+
Cheesy Italian shells	½ c	160	1	Na	0.5	1	6	0	2	0	+
Chili macaroni	⅓ c	140	1	Na	0	1	3	0	2	0	+
Italian sausage	⅓ c	130	0.5	Na	0	1	5	0	0	0	+
Lasagna	⅔ c	120	0.5	0	0	1	5	0	0	0	+
Philly cheese steak	½ c	140	3.5	Na	1.5	1	2	0	0	0	+
Salisbury	½ c	120	0.5	0	0	1	1	0	0	0	+

Food	Portion Size	Calories	Total Fat (g)	Good Fats (g)	Bad Fats (g)	Fiber (g)	Sugars (mg)	Beta-carotene (mcg)	Calcium (%DV)	Vit. C (%DV)	B vit. (0,+,++)
Stroganoff	½ c	130	1	0	0	1	3	0	2	0	+
Tomato basil penne	⅓ c	140	0.5	0	0	1	6	0	0	0	+
HEALTH BARS AND SHAKES											
Atkins Advantage											
Almond brownie bar	1	220	9	Na	4	7	0	Na	25	25	+
Chocolate coconut bar	1	230	10	Na	8	10	3	Na	30	25	+
Chocolate peanut butter	1	240	11	Na	6	10	1	Na	30	25	+
Atkins Morning Start											
Apple crisp bar	1	180	9	Na	4.5	7	1	Na	40	15	+
Chocolate chip bar	1	180	7	Na	3.5	5	1	Na	20	15	+
Mixed berry bar	1	150	5	Na	1	4	1	Na	25	15	+
Oatmeal raisin bar	1	140	5	Na	2	5	3	Na	35	15	+
Strawberry crisp bar	1	160	9	Na	4.5	7	1	Na	40	15	+
Balance Bar											
Almond brownie, original	1	200	6	Na	1.5	2	18	Na	10	100	‡
Chocolate, original	1	200	6	Na	3.5	<1	18	Na	10	100	‡
Cookie dough, original	1	200	6	Na	3.5	<1	18	Na	10	100	‡
Mocha chip, original	1	200	6	Na	3.5	<1	19	Na	10	100	‡
Clif Bar											
Blueberry crisp	1	240	5	Na	0.5	5	21	Na	25	100	+
Carrot cake	1	240	4	Na	1.5	5	21	Na	25	100	+
Chocolate chip	1	250	5	Na	2	5	21	Na	25	100	+
Lemon poppy seed	1	240	3.5	Na	1.5	5	21	Na	25	100	+
Oatmeal raisin walnut	1	240	5	Na	1	5	20	Na	25	100	+

Food	Portion Size	Calories	Total Fat (g)	Good Fats (g)	Bad Fats (g)	Fiber (g)	Sugars (mg)	Beta-carotene (mcg)	Calcium (%DV)	Vit. C (%DV)	B vit. (0,+,++)
Luna											
Caramel nut brownie	1	190	6	Na	3	4	11	Na	35	100	‡
Chocolate peppermint stick	1	180	5	Na	2.5	3	9	Na	35	100	‡‡
Key lime pie	1	180	4	Na	3	3	10	Na	180	35	‡‡
Lemon zest	1	180	4	Na	3	3	10	Na	35	100	‡‡
S'mores	1	180	5	Na	3	3	9	Na	35	100	‡
Power Bar, Harvest Whole Grain											
Dipped double chocolate crisp	1	250	5	Na	2.5	5	20	Na	40	80	‡‡
Dipped oatmeal raisin	1	250	5	Na	2	5	22	Na	40	80	‡‡
Heart healthy apple cinnamon crisp	1	240	4	Na	0.5	5	20	Na	40	80	‡‡
Heart healthy strawberry crunch	1	240	4	Na	0.5	5	20	Na	40	80	‡
Power Bar Performance											
Apple cinnamon	1	230	2.5	Na	0	2	24	Na	35	100	‡‡
Banana	1	230	2.5	Na	0	2	20	Na	35	100	‡‡
Chocolate peanut butter	1	240	3	Na	0.5	2	23	Na	35	100	‡‡
Oatmeal raisin	1	230	2	Na	0	2	25	Na	35	100	‡‡
Wild berry	1	230	2	Na	0	2	24	Na	35	100	‡
Power Bar Pria 110 Plus											
Chocolate peanut crunch	1	110	3.5	Na	2	1	10	Na	30	60	‡
Double chocolate cookie	1	110	3	Na	2.5	1	10	Na	30	60	‡‡
French vanilla crisp	1	110	3	Na	2.5	1	9	Na	30	60	‡‡
PowerBar Protein Plus											
Chocolate crisp	1	290	6	Na	3.5	2	18	Na	45	100	‡‡
Chocolate peanut butter	1	300	6	Na	3.5	1	19	Na	40	100	‡‡

Food	Portion Size	Calories	Total Fat (g)	Good Fats (g)	Bad Fats (g)	Fiber (g)	Sugars (mg)	Beta-carotene (mcg)	Calcium (%DV)	Vit. C (%DV)	B vit. (0,+,++)
Cookies & cream	1	300	6	Na	3.5	1	18	Na	40	100	++
Vanilla yogurt	1	300	6	Na	3.5	1	19	Na	45	100	++
PowerBar Triple Threat											
Caramel peanut fusion	1	230	8	Na	4.5	4	15	Na	15	100	++
Caramel peanut crisp	1	220	5	Na	2	4	14	Na	15	100	++
Chocolate caramel	1	230	8	Na	4.5	4	15	Na	15	100	++
Chocolate peanut butter crisp	1	220	5	Na	2	4	14	Na	15	100	++
Slim Fast Optima Meal Bars											
Blueberry crisp	1	180	4	Na	2.5	3	12	Na	25	35	+
Chocolate chip granola	1	220	6	Na	3.5	2	15	Na	30	35	+
Milk chocolate peanut	1	220	5	Na	3	3	14	Na	30	35	+
Rich chocolate brownie	1	220	5	Na	3.5	2	15	Na	30	35	+
Strawberry cheesecake	1	220	6	Na	4	2	13	Na	30	35	+
Trail mix chewy granola	1	210	5	Na	1	2	15	Na	30	35	+
Slim Fast Optima Shakes											
Cappuccino delight, can	1	180	6	3.5	2	5	18	Na	50	100	+
French vanilla, can	1	180	6	2.5	2.5	5	17	Na	50	100	+
Rich chocolate royale, can	1	190	6	3	2.5	5	18	Na	50	100	+
Strawberry 'n cream, can	1	180	5	2.5	2	5	17	Na	50	100	+
Slim Fast Optima Snack Bars											
Apple cinnamon muffin	1	140	5	3	0.5	1	9	Na	25	0	+
Banana & nut muffin	1	150	8	4.5	0.5	1	6	Na	25	0	+
Blueberry muffin	1	140	5	3	0.5	1	9	Na	25	0	+
Chocolate mint crisp	1	120	4	Na	3	<1	7	Na	25	15	+

Food	Portion Size	Calories	Total Fat (g)	Good Fats (g)	Bad Fats (g)	Fiber (g)	Sugars (mg)	Beta-carotene (mcg)	Calcium (%DV)	Vit. C (%DV)	B vit. (0,+,++)
Crispy peanut caramel	1	120	4	Na	3	1	8	Na	25	15	+
Oatmeal raisin cookie	1	120	3.5	Na	1.5	1	8	Na	25	0	+
Peanut butter crunch	1	120	4	Na	2	<1	12	Na	2	0	+
HERRING, Atlantic, kippered	1 oz	61	3	1.5	1	0	0	Na	2	0	+
Atlantic, pickled	1 oz	74	5	Na	1	0	0	Na	2	0	+
Pacific, broiled	3 oz	212	15	7.5	4	0	0	Na	9	0	+
HONEY	1 tbs	64	0	0	0	0	17	0	1	0	0
HONEYDEW, raw, balls	1 c	64	0	0	0	1	14	53	1	53	0
HORSERADISH, prep.	1 tbs	7	0	0	0	0	1	0	0	6	0
HUMMUS											
Athenos, artichoke & garlic; black olive; cucumber dill; original; roasted garlic	2 tbs	50	3	0.5*	0	<1	<1	0	0	2	0
Athenos, roasted eggplant	2 tbs	45	3	0.5*	0	<1	<1	0	0	2	0
Athenos, roasted red pepper	2 tbs	50	3	0.5*	0	<1	<1	0	0	15	0
Fantastic Foods	2 tbs	60	2	Na	0	2	0	0	2	0	0
ICE CREAM											
Ben & Jerry's											
Black & tan	½ c	230	13	Na	9	1	21	Na	15	0	0
Butter pecan	½ c	280	21	Na	10	0	18	Na	15	0	0
Cherry Garcia	½ c	250	14	Na	10	<1	22	Na	15	0	0
Chocolate	½ c	260	16	Na	11	2	28	Na	15	0	0
Chunky monkey	½ c	300	18	Na	10	1	28	Na	15	2	0
Coffee	½ c	240	15	Na	10	0	19	Na	15	0	0

Food	Portion Size	Calories	Total Fat (g)	Good Fats (g)	Bad Fats (g)	Fiber (g)	Sugars (mg)	Beta-carotene (mcg)	Calcium (%DV)	Vit. C (%DV)	B vit. (0,+,++)
Fossil fuel	½ c	280	18	Na	12	1	26	Na	15	0	0
Half-baked	½ c	280	14	Na	9	<1	26	Na	10	0	0
Mint chocolate cookie	½ c	260	16	Na	9	0	21	Na	15	0	0
NY Super fudge chunk	½ c	310	20	Na	11	2	25	Na	15	0	0
Neopolitan dynamite	½ c	250	13	Na	9	1	26	Na	10	0	0
Turtle soup	½ c	280	15	Na	10	1	25	Na	15	0	0
Vanilla Heath bar crunch	½ c	290	18	Na	12	0	27	Na	15	0	0
Vermonty python	½ c	310	19	Na	11	1	26	Na	5	0	0
Breyers											
Butter pecan, no sugar added	½ c	122	7	Na	4	1	4	0	8	1	0
Cherry vanilla	½ c	140	6	Na	4	0	16	Na	10	0	0
Chocolate	½ c	140	7	Na	4.5	1	16	Na	8	0	0
Cookies & cream, natural	½ c	160	8	Na	5	0	16	Na	10	0	0
French vanilla	½ c	150	8	Na	4.5	0	15	Na	10	0	0
Mint chocolate chip, natural	½ c	160	8	Na	6	1	16	Na	10	0	0
Rocky road	½ c	160	9	Na	5	1	17	Na	8	0	0
Strawberry	½ c	120	5	Na	3.5	0	15	Na	8	10	0
Dreyer's											
Almond praline	½ c	150	7	Na	4	0	16	Na	4	0	0
Butter pecan	½ c	170	10	Na	4.5	0	13	Na	6	0	0
Chocolate	½ c	150	8	Na	4.5	1	15	Na	6	0	0
Cookie dough	½ c	180	9	Na	6	0	15	Na	6	0	0
Fudge tracks	½ c	180	11	Na	6	0	16	Na	6	0	0

Food	Portion Size	Calories	Total Fat (g)	Good Fats (g)	Bad Fats (g)	Fiber (g)	Sugars (mg)	Beta-carotene (mcg)	Calcium (%DV)	Vit. C (%DV)	B vit. (0,+,++)
Mocha almond fudge	½ c	180	11	Na	6	0	16	Na	6	0	0
Peanut butter cup	½ c	180	10	Na	4	0	15	Na	6	0	0
Rocky road	½ c	170	10	Na	5	1	14	Na	6	0	0
Spumoni	½ c	150	8	Na	4.5	0	13	Na	6	0	0
Toffee bar crunch	½ c	160	8	Na	5	0	19	Na	6	0	0
Dreyer's—Slow Churned Light											
Butter pecan	½ c	120	5	Na	2	0	12	Na	6	0	0
Chocolate chip	½ c	120	4.5	Na	3	0	13	Na	6	0	0
Cookies & cream	½ c	120	4	Na	2	0	13	Na	6	0	0
Mint chocolate chip	½ c	120	4.5	Na	3	0	13	Na	6	0	0
Rocky road	½ c	120	4	Na	2	0	12	Na	6	0	0
Strawberry	½ c	110	3	Na	1.5	0	13	Na	6	0	0
Vanilla bean	½ c	100	3.5	Na	2	0	11	Na	6	0	0
Vanilla chocolate	½ c	100	3.5	Na	2	0	11	Na	6	0	0
Häagen-Dazs—Regular											
Bailey's Irish Cream	½ c	270	17	Na	10.5	0	22	Na	15	0	0
Banana split	½ c	280	16	Na	9	0	27	Na	10	2	0
Black walnut	½ c	300	22	Na	11.5	0	19	Na	10	0	0
Butter pecan	½ c	310	23	Na	11.5	<1	18	Na	15	0	0
Cherry vanilla	½ c	240	15	Na	9.5	0	22	Na	10	2	0
Chocolate	½ c	270	18	Na	11.5	1	21	Na	15	0	0
Chocolate peanut butter	½ c	360	24	Na	11	2	24	Na	10	0	0
English toffee	½ c	350	22	Na	13.5	0	31	Na	10	0	0
Rocky road	½ c	300	18	Na	9	1	24	Na	10	0	0

Food	Portion Size	Calories	Total Fat (g)	Good Fats (g)	Bad Fats (g)	Fiber (g)	Sugars (mg)	Beta-carotene (mcg)	Calcium (%DV)	Vit. C (%DV)	B vit. (0, +, ++)
Häagen-Dazs–Light											
Blueberry cheesecake	½ c	230	7	Na	4.5	0	28	Na	10	0	0
Cherry fudge truffle	½ c	230	7	Na	4	0	33	Na	10	0	0
Mint chip	½ c	230	8	Na	5	0	30	Na	15	0	0
Vanilla caramel brownie	½ c	240	7	Na	4	0	31	Na	15	0	0
ICE CREAM NOVELTIES											
Dreyer's											
Dibs, caramel w/chocolate coating	26 pcs	440	32	Na	22	1	28	Na	10	0	0
Dibs, cookies & cream w/chocolate coating	26 pcs	410	29	Na	20	1	23	Na	10	0	0
Dibs, peanut butter w/chocolate coating	26 pcs	510	39	Na	23	2	23	Na	8	0	0
Dibs, vanilla w/chocolate coating	26 pcs	420	28	Na	20	0	24	Na	8	0	0
Dibs, vanilla w/Nestle Crunch	26 pcs	380	28	Na	20	0	24	0	8	0	0
Fruit bars: grape	1	80	0	0	0	0	20	Na	0	0	0
Fruit bars: orange & cream	1	80	1.5	0	0.5	0	15	Na	4	0	0
Fruit bars: strawberry	1	80	0	0	0	1	20	Na	0	0	0
Good Humor											
Chocolate éclair bar	1	230	11	Na	4.5	1	16	Na	4	0	0
Cone, Oreo cookies & cream	1	220	10	Na	6	1	20	Na	6	0	0
Cone, premium sundae	1	260	15	Na	9	1	18	Na	6	0	0
Cyclone cookies & cream	1	380	20	Na	10.5	1	35	Na	15	0	0
Strawberry shortcake bar	1	230	12	Na	6.5	1	18	Na	4	0	0
Toasted almond bar	1	240	12	Na	6	1	23	Na	6	0	0

Food	Portion Size	Calories	Total Fat (g)	Good Fats (g)	Bad Fats (g)	Fiber (g)	Sugars (mg)	Beta-carotene (mcg)	Calcium (%DV)	Vit. C (%DV)	B vit. (0,+,++)
Häagen-Dazs											
Chocolate & dark chocolate bar	1	300	21	Na	13	<1	21	Na	8	0	0
Coffee & almond crunch bar	1	310	22	Na	12	<1	21	Na	10	0	0
Mint & dark chocolate bar	1	290	20	Na	12	1	20	Na	8	0	0
Vanilla & milk chocolate bar	1	290	21	Na	14	0	21	Na	8	0	0
Klondike											
Bar, chocolate	4.5 oz	250	17	Na	13	1	18	Na	8	0	0
Bar, Heath	4.5 oz	250	17	Na	13	0	19	Na	8	0	0
Bar, Krunch	4 oz	460	17	Na	12	0	19	Na	8	0	0
Bar, Oreo	4 oz	260	17	Na	11	1	19	Na	6	0	0
Bar, Reese's	4 oz	270	18	Na	11	1	20	Na	8	0	0
Bar, vanilla	4.5 oz	250	17	Na	13	0	18	Na	8	0	0
Cone, vanilla	4.3 oz	280	16	Na	9	1	20	Na	8	0	0
Sandwich, ice cream cookie	1	260	12	Na	7	1	22	Na	4	0	0
Sandwich, vanilla	1	180	6	Na	4	0	16	Na	6	0	0
Popsicle											
Creamsicle	1.65 oz	70	1	0	0.5	0	8	Na	4	10	0
Creamsicle, sugar free	1	40	2	0	1.5	6	0	Na	2	0	0
Fudgsicle	1.65 oz	60	1.5	0	1.5	0	9	Na	10	0	0
ICE CREAM SUBSTITUTES (non-dairy)											
Soy Delicious—Organic											
Butter pecan	½ c	160	7	Na	1	3	12	Na	0	0	0
Chocolate velvet	½ c	130	3.5	Na	0.5	1	14	Na	0	0	0

162

Food	Portion Size	Calories	Total Fat (g)	Good Fats (g)	Bad Fats (g)	Fiber (g)	Sugars (mg)	Beta-carotene (mcg)	Calcium (%DV)	Vit. C (%DV)	B vit. (0-+-++)
Creamy vanilla	½ c	130	3	Na	0	3	13	Na	0	0	0
Mocha fudge	½ c	130	3	Na	0	3	15	Na	0	0	0
Peanut butter	½ c	150	6	Na	1	3	12	Na	0	0	0
Soy Delicious—Novelties											
Li'l Buddies, chocolate	1	150	3	Na	1	2	12	Na	0	0	0
Li'l Buddies, vanilla	1	150	3	Na	1	2	13	Na	0	0	0
So Delicious Dairy-Free bars, orange	1	80	5	Na	0	2	12	Na	10	0	0
So Delicious Dairy-Free bars fudge	1	90	3	Na	0	2	9	Na	0	0	0
Sweet Nothings, fudge bar	1	100	0	0	0	0	12	Na	0	8	0
Sweet Nothings, mango raspberry	1	100	0	0	0	0	12	Na	0	8	0
JAM, JELLY, PRESERVES											
Cascadian Farm Fruit Spreads, all flavors	1 tbs	40	0	0	0	0	10	0	0	0	0
Smuckers jam, all flavors	1 tbs	50	0	0	0	0	12	0	0	0	0
Smuckers jelly, all flavors	1 tbs	50	0	0	0	0	12	0	0	0	0
Smuckers preserves, all flavors	1 tbs	50	0	0	0	0	12	0	0	0	0
KALE, fresh, cooked, chopped, no salt	1 c	36	1	0	0	3	2	10,625	4	88	0
KETCHUP											
Del Monte	1 tbs	15	0	0	0	0	4	0	0	0	0
Hunts	1 tbs	15	0	0	0	0	4	0	0	0	0
KIELBASA											
Hillshire, Polska	2 oz	180	15	Na	6	0	0	0	0	1	0
Jennie-O, turkey	2 oz	70	3	Na	1	0	1	0	2	0	0
Oscar Mayer, Polska, turkey	2 oz	90	5	Na	1.5	0	1	0	0	0	0

Food	Portion Size	Calories	Total Fat (g)	Good Fats (g)	Bad Fats (g)	Fiber (g)	Sugars (mg)	Beta-carotene (mcg)	Calcium (%DV)	Vit. C (%DV)	B vit. (0,+,++)
KUMQUAT, raw	1	13	0	0	0	1	2	0	1	13	0
LAMB											
Australian, sirloin chop, lean, broiled	3 oz	160	7	3	3	0	0	0	1	0	+
Australian, leg, whole, lean, roasted	3 oz	162	7	3	3	0	0	0	0	0	++
Australian shoulder blade, lean & fat, broiled	3 oz	247	19	6	9	0	0	0	2	0	++
Domestic, leg, sirloin half, lean & fat, roasted	3 oz	241	17	7	7	0	0	0	0	0	+++
Domestic, loin, lean, roasted	3 oz	172	8	3	3	0	0	0	1	0	+++
Domestic, rib, lean & fat, roasted	3 oz	290	23	10	10	0	0	0	1	0	+++
NZ, frozen, loin, lean & fat, broiled	3 oz	252	18	7	9	0	0	0	1	0	+++
NZ, frozen, rib, lean, roasted	3 oz	167	9	3.5	4	0	0	0	1	0	++
NZ, frozen, shoulder, lean & fat, braised	3 oz	291	20	8	10	0	0	0	2	0	+
LEMON, raw, peeled	1 c	61	1	0	0	6	5	6	5	181	0
LEMONADE											
Country Time, regular or pink	8 oz	60	0	0	0	0	16	0	0	10	0
Country Time, strawberry	8 oz	80	0	0	0	0	20	0	0	0	0
Minute Maid, frozen, country	8 oz	110	0	0	0	0	27	0	0	15	0
Minute Maid, carton	8 oz	110	0	0	0	0	29	0	0	0	0
Minute Maid, raspberry, carton	8 oz	120	0	0	0	0	30	0	0	0	+
LENTILS, cooked, no salt	1 c	230	1	0	0	16	4	10	3	4	+
LETTUCE											
Butterhead (Boston, bibb), shredded	1 c	7	0	0	0	1	1	1092	1	3	0
Green leaf, shredded	1 c	5	0	0	0	0	0	1600	1	10	0
Iceberg, shredded	1 c	8	0	0	0	1	1	215	1	3	0

Food	Portion Size	Calories	Total Fat (g)	Good Fats (g)	Bad Fats (g)	Fiber (g)	Sugars (mg)	Beta-carotene (mcg)	Calcium (%DV)	Vit. C (%DV)	B vit. (0,+,++)
Red leaf, shredded	1 c	4	0	0	0	0	0	1258	0	1	0
Romaine, shredded	1 c	8	0	0	0	1	1	1637	1	18	0
LIMA BEANS, fresh, boiled, no salt	1 c	209	1	0	0	13	6	0	3	0	+
Birds Eye (frozen), baby limas, cooked	½ c	110	0	0	0	5	0	0	4	15	+
Birds Eye (frozen), Fordhook	½ c	100	0	0	0	4	0	0	0	25	+
Del Monte, canned	½ c	80	0	0	0	4	0	0	2	8	+
Green Giant, baby limas & butter, cooked	⅔ c	100	1.5	0	1	5	1	0	2	15	+
LIME, fresh	1	20	0	0	0	2	1	20	2	32	0
LIVER (see beef, chicken, duck)											
LIVERWURST											
LOBSTER											
Northern, cooked	1 oz	91	8	Na	3	0	0	0	0	0	+
Spiny	3 oz	83	1	Na	0	0	0	0	5	0	0
LUNCHABLES	3 oz	122	2	Na	0	0	0	0	5	2	+
Bologna & American cracker stackers	1 pkg	390	22	Na	10	1	12	0	25	0	0
Chicken dunks	1 pkg	310	6	Na	2	0	35	0	2	20	0
Chicken shakeups BBQ	1 pkg	220	6	Na	2	1	16	0	15	100	0
Chicken strips, maxed out	1 pkg	480	15	Na	4.5	1	32	0	6	20	0
Ham & cheese cracker stackers	1 pkg	400	20	Na	10	1	14	0	20	0	0
Ham & Swiss	1 pkg	340	17	Na	10	1	6	0	35	0	0
Ham & Swiss, low fat, cracker stackers	1 pkg	330	9	Na	4.5	1	30	0	35	100	0
Mini burgers, grilled	1 pkg	390	11	Na	5.5	1	34	0	20	100	0
Nachos	1 pkg	380	21	Na	6	1	3	0	0	0	0
Pizza stix, maxed out	1 pkg	680	10	Na	4.5	3	72	0	40	25	0

165

Food	Portion Size	Calories	Total Fat (g)	Good Fats (g)	Bad Fats (g)	Fiber (g)	Sugars (mg)	Beta-carotene (mcg)	Calcium (%DV)	Vit. C (%DV)	B vit. (0,+,++)
Pizza & Treatza	1 pkg	460	10	Na	4.5	4	46	0	35	4	0
Taco beef	1 pkg	450	10	Na	4.5	1	34	0	50	2	0
Turkey & American cracker stackers	1 pkg	420	17	Na	8.5	1	39	0	25	100	0
Turkey, ham, swiss, cheddar	1 pkg	360	19	Na	10	1	8	0	30	0	0
LUNCHEON LOAF											
Oscar Mayer, ham & cheese	1 oz	60	4.5	2	2.5	0	1	0	1	0	0
Oscar Mayer, luncheon loaf spiced	1 oz	60	4.5	2	1.5	0	1	0	3	0	0
Oscar Mayer, olive loaf	1 oz	80	6	3	2	0	1	0	3	0	0
Oscar Mayer, pickle & pimento loaf	1 oz	80	6	3	2	0	2	0	3	0	0
MACADAMIA NUTS,											
dry roasted, no salt	1 oz	203	21	16.5	3	2	1	0	1	0	0
MACARONI (Also see "Pasta")											
MACARONI & CHEESE (boxed, mix)											
(Also see "Pasta" and "Frozen Dinners")											
Kraft Deluxe w/original cheddar cheese	3.5 oz	320	10	Na	3.5	2	4	Na	15	0	Na
Kraft Deluxe sharp cheddar	3.5 oz	320	10	Na	3.5	1	4	Na	15	0	Na
Kraft Dinner Deluxe ½ the fat	3.5 oz	290	4.5	Na	2.5	1	6	Na	20	0	Na
Kraft Dinner Deluxe 4 cheese sauce	3.5 oz	320	10	Na	3.5	3	5	Na	15	0	Na
Kraft Premium cheesy alfredo	2 oz	260	2.5	Na	1	2	8	Na	10	0	Na
Kraft Premium thick 'n creamy	2 oz	250	2	Na	1	2	8	Na	10	0	Na
Kraft Premium three cheese	2 oz	260	2.5	Na	1	2	7	Na	10	0	Na
Kraft The Cheesiest	2 oz	260	2.5	Na	1	1	7	Na	20	0	Na

Food	Portion Size	Calories	Total Fat (g)	Good Fats (g)	Bad Fats (g)	Fiber (g)	Sugars (mg)	Beta-carotene (mcg)	Calcium (%DV)	Vit. C (%DV)	B vit. (0,+,++)
MACKEREL											
Atlantic, broiled	3 oz	223	15	6	4	0	0	0	1	0	‡‡
King, broiled	3 oz	114	2	1	0	0	0	0	3	2	‡‡
Pacific, broiled	3 oz	171	9	3	2	0	0	0	2	2	‡‡
Spanish, broiled	3 oz	134	5	2	2	0	0	0	1	2	‡‡
w/tomato sauce (Chicken of the Sea)	3 oz	70	3	1	1	0	1	0	15	0	+
MANGO, fresh, sliced	1 c	107	0	0	0	3	24	734	1	76	0
MARGARINE & SPREADS											
Benecol, regular	1 tbs	70	8	4.5	1	0	0	0	0	0	0
Benecol, light	1 tbs	50	5	2.5	0.5	0	0	0	0	0	0
Blue Bonnet, regular stick	1 tbs	80	9	2.5	3.5	0	0	0	0	0	0
Blue Bonnet, light stick	1 tbs	50	5	1.5	1.5	0	0	0	0	0	0
Blue Bonnet homestyle soft	1 tbs	60	7	1.5	1	0	0	0	0	0	0
Blue Bonnet homestyle light, soft	1 tbs	40	4.5	Na	1	0	0	0	0	0	0
Country Crock, regular, tub & sticks	1 tbs	60	7	1.5	2.5	0	0	0	0	0	0
Country Crock, churn style	1 tbs	80	8	2.5	3	0	0	0	0	0	0
Country Crock, light	1 tbs	50	5	1.5	1.5	0	0	0	0	0	0
Country Crock plus calcium	1 tbs	50	5	1.5	1.5	0	0	0	10	0	0
I Can't Believe It's Not Butter, fat free	1 tbs	5	0	0	0	0	0	0	0	0	+
I Can't Believe It's Not Butter, light, soft	1 tbs	50	5	1.5	1	0	0	Na	0	0	+
I Can't Believe It's Not Butter, orig., soft	1 tbs	80	8	2	2	0	0	Na	0	0	0
I Can't Believe It's Not Butter, spray	5 sprays	0	0	0	0	0	0	0	0	0	0
Parkay, light, tub	1 tbs	50	5	1.5	1	0	0	0	0	0	0
Parkay, orig. stick	1 tbs	80	9	3	3	0	0	Na	0	0	+

Food	Portion Size	Calories	Total Fat (g)	Good Fats (g)	Bad Fats (g)	Fiber (g)	Sugars (mg)	Beta-carotene (mcg)	Calcium (%DV)	Vit. C (%DV)	B vit. (0,+,++)
Parkay, soft tub	1 tbs	60	7	2	1.5	0	0	Na	0	0	+
Promise buttery spread, soft, light	1 tbs	45	5	1.5	1	0	0	Na	0	0	+
Promise buttery spread, soft	1 tbs	80	8	3	1.5	0	0	Na	0	0	+
Smart Balance, 67% light spread	1 tbs	80	9	3.5	2.5	0	0	Na	0	0	+
Smart Balance, 37% light spread	1 tbs	45	5	2	1.5	0	0	Na	0	0	+
Smart Balance Omega Plus	1 tbs	80	9	3.5	2.5	0	0	Na	0	0	+
MARSHMALLOWS											
Jet-puffed creme	2 tbs	40	0	0	0	0	8	0	0	0	0
Jet-puffed, funmallows	4 pcs	110	0	0	0	0	18	0	0	0	0
Jet-puffed, toasted coconut	3 pcs	100	2.5	Na	2	0	16	0	0	0	0
MAYONNAISE & SALAD DRESSING											
Hellman's canola	1 tbs	90	10	5	1	0	0	0	0	0	0
Hellman's light	1 tbs	45	4.5	Na	0.5	0	0	0	0	0	0
Kraft, fat free	1 tbs	10	0	0	0	0	0	0	0	0	0
Kraft, real mayonnaise	1 tbs	100	11	Na	2	0	1	0	0	0	0
Miracle Whip, fat free	1 tbs	15	0	0	0	0	2	0	0	0	0
Miracle Whip, light	1 tbs	25	1.5	Na	0	0	2	0	0	0	0
Miracle Whip, orig. dressing	1 tbs	40	3.5	Na	0.5	0	2	0	0	0	0
MILK											
1% protein fortified	1 c	118	3	0.5	2	0	0	0	34	4	+
2% protein fortified	1 c	138	5	1.5	3	0	13	7	35	4	+
Buttermilk, low fat	1 c	98	2	0.5	1	0	12	2	28	4	+
Evaporated, non-fat	½ c	100	0	0	0	0	15	0	37	2	+
Evaporated, whole	½ c	169	10	3	6	0	0	0	32	3	+

Food	Portion Size	Calories	Total Fat (g)	Good Fats (g)	Bad Fats (g)	Fiber (g)	Sugars (mg)	Beta-carotene (mcg)	Calcium (%DV)	Vit. C (%DV)	B vit. (0,+,++)
Lactaid, fat free	1 c	80	0	Na	0	0	12	0	30	0	+
Lactaid, 2%	1 c	130	5	Na	3	0	12	0	30	0	+
Skim, calcium fortified	1 c	86	0	0	0	0	12	0	50	4	+
Whole	1 c	146	8	2	4.5	0	13	12	27	0	+
MIXED FRUIT											
Del Monte, cherry mixed	½ c	90	0	0	0	<1	19	150*	0	8	0
Del Monte, chunky mixed	½ c	100	0	0	0	1	23	150*	0	4	0
Del Monte, fruit cocktail	½ c	100	0	0	0	1	23	150*	0	4	0
Dole, mixed, frozen	¾ c	60	0	0	0	2	12	Na	0	160	0
Dole, tropical mixed	½ c	90	0	0	0	1	20	Na	0	45	0
S&W, chunky mixed, natural style	½ c	80	0	0	0	3	16	175*	0	2	0
S&W, cocktail, lite syrup	½ c	70	0	0	0	1	16	175*	0	2	0
MOLASSES, blackstrap	1 tbs	47	0	0	0	0	0	0	17	0	
Regular	1 tbs	58	0	0	0	0	11	0	4	0	
MUFFINS (box/pouch mixes only)											
Betty Crocker											
Apple streusel	¼ c mix	160	3	Na	1.5	1	17	Na	0	0	0
Banana nut	3 tbs	150	3.5	Na	1	<1	13	Na	0	0	0
Chocolate chip, pouch	⅕ pkg	160	5	Na	3	1	14	Na	0	0	0
Cinnamon streusel	1/12 pkg	150	3.5	Na	2	0	17	Na	0	0	0
Double chocolate	1/12 pkg	190	7	2	4	0	20	Na	20	0	0
Lemon poppy seed	1/12 pkg	140	2	Na	1	0	19	Na	2	0	0
Lemon poppy seed, pouch	⅙ pkg	130	3.5	Na	2	0	12	Na	0	0	0

Food	Portion Size	Calories	Total Fat (g)	Good Fats (g)	Bad Fats (g)	Fiber (g)	Sugars (mg)	Beta-carotene (mcg)	Calcium (%DV)	Vit. C (%DV)	B vit. (0,+,++)
Twice the blueberries	¼ c mix	120	1	0	0	1	17	Na	0	2	0
Wild blueberry	½2 pkg	130	1.5	Na	0.5	<1	15	Na	0	0	0
Jiffy											
Apple cinnamon, mix	¼ c	160	6	Na	2	0	12	Na	4	0	0
Banana nut, mix	¼ c	150	6	Na	2	<1	10	Na	4	0	0
Blueberry, mix	¼ c	160	5	Na	2	0	11	Na	4	0	0
Bran, mix	¼ c	140	4.5	Na	1.5	2	9	Na	4	0	0
Raspberry, mix	¼ c	160	6	Na	2	0	11	Na	4	0	0
MUSHROOMS											
Brown or Italian, raw	1 oz	6	0	0	0	0	0	0	0	0	0
Green Giant, canned, whole or slices	½ c	25	0	0	0	1	1	0	0	0	0
Portobello, raw, diced	1 c	22	0	0	0	2	2	0	0	0	+
Shiitake, cooked, no salt	1 c	81	0	0	0	3	6	0	0	0	+
MUSSELS											
Blue, cooked	3 oz	146	4	Na	1	0	0	0	2	19	‡
Gold seal, in cottonseed oil, whole, smoked	2 oz	4	Na	1.5	0	0	0	0	4	0	‡
MUSTARD											
Grey Poupon, country Dijon	1 tsp	5	0	0	0	0	0	0	0	0	0
Grey Poupon, honey mustard	1 tsp	10	0	0	0	0	0	0	0	0	0
Yellow, prepared	1 tsp	3	0	0	0	0	0	0	0	0	0
MUSTARD GREENS, cooked, chopped	1 c	21	0	0	0	3	0	5311	10	54	0

Food	Portion Size	Calories	Total Fat (g)	Good Fats (g)	Bad Fats (g)	Fiber (g)	Sugars (mg)	Beta-carotene (mcg)	Calcium (%DV)	Vit. C (%DV)	B vit. (0,+,++)
NECTARINE, 2.5" diameter	1	60	0	0	0	2	11	204	0	12	0
NOODLES (dry)											
Egg, cooked, enriched	1 c	212	2	0.5	0.5	2	0	0	1	0	+
Egg, spinach, cooked, enriched	1 c	211	3	0.5	1	4	1	81	3	0	+
Japanese, soba, cooked	1 c	112	0	0	0	0	0	0	0	0	0
OCEAN PERCH, Atlantic, broiled	3 oz	103	2	0.5	0	0	0	0	11	1	+
OILS											
Almond	1 tbs	120	13	9	1	0	0	0	0	0	0
Canola	1 tbs	120	14	9	1	0	0	0	0	0	0
Corn	1 tbs	120	14	4	2	0	0	0	0	0	0
Corn & canola (Mazola Right Blend)	1 tbs	120	14	8	1	0	0	0	0	0	0
Olive	1 tbs	120	14	10	2	0	0	0	0	0	0
Sesame	1 tbs	120	14	5	2	0	0	0	0	0	0
Soybean	1 tbs	120	13	9	2	0	0	0	0	0	0
OLIVES											
Lindsay, black, large	4	25	2.5	1.5	0	0	0	36*	0	0	0
Lindsay, green, medium	5	25	2.5	1.5	0	0	0	40*	0	0	0
Lindsay, green, slices w/pimentos	2 tbs	25	2.5	1.5	0	0	0	40*	0	0	0
Lindsay, kalamata	3	25	2.5	2	0	0	0	36*	0	0	0
ONIONS											
Fresh, chopped, yellow or red	1 c	67	0	0	0	2	7	1.6	3	17	0
Fresh, tops and bulbs (scallions)	1 c	32	0	0	0	3	2	598	7	31	0
Nathans, frozen, rings	6 pcs	200	10	Na	4	1	5	Na	0	4	0

Food	Portion Size	Calories	Total Fat (g)	Good Fats (g)	Bad Fats (g)	Fiber (g)	Sugars (mg)	Beta-carotene (mcg)	Calcium (%DV)	Vit. C (%DV)	B vit. (0,+,++)
ORANGES											
Fresh, California, 2 5/8" dia.	1	59	0	0	0	3	0	0	4	97	0
Fresh, Florida, 2 5/8" dia.	1	65	0	0	0	3	13	100	6	105	0
Mandarin, canned (Dole)	½ c	80	0	0	0	1	18	Na	0	35	0
ORANGE JUICE/BEVERAGE											
Cascadian Farm, frozen, organic	8 oz	110	0	0	0	0	26	Na	0	130	0
Minute Maid, country style, carton	8 oz	110	0	0	0	0	24	Na	2	120	+
Minute Maid, homestyle w/calcium & vit. D	8 oz	110	0	0	0	0	24	Na	35	120	+
Minute Maid, orange passion, carton	8 oz	130	0	0	0	0	29	Na	35	120	+
Tang, prep.	8 oz	90	0	0	0	0	23	0	9	100	0
Tang, orange pineapple, prep.	8 oz	100	0	0	0	0	24	0	6	100	0
Tropicana, calcium & vitamin D	8 oz	110	0	0	0	0	22	Na	35	120	+
Tropicana, Essentials Light 'n Healthy w/calcium	8 oz	50	0	0	0	0	10	Na	20	120	+
Tropicana, Essentials Fiber	8 oz	120	0	0	0	3	22	Na	2	120	+
Tropicana, original, no pulp	8 oz	110	0	0	0	0	22	Na	2	120	+
OYSTERS											
Canned	3 oz	58	2	Na	1	0	0	0	3	7	+
Eastern, raw, wild	1 c	169	6	1	2	0	0	0	11	15	++
Pacific, raw	3 oz	69	2	Na	0	0	0	0	0	11	+
PANCAKE/WAFFLE (mix, unprep.)											
Aunt Jemima, buckwheat	¼ c	100	1	Na	1	3	3	0	4	0	0
Aunt Jemima, buttermilk complete	⅓ c	160	2	Na	0.5	1	6	0	15	0	+
Aunt Jemima, original	⅓ c	150	0.5	0	0	1	7	0	10	0	+

Food	Portion Size	Calories	Total Fat (g)	Good Fats (g)	Bad Fats (g)	Fiber (g)	Sugars (mg)	Beta-carotene (mcg)	Calcium (%DV)	Vit. C (%DV)	B vit. (0,+,++)
Aunt Jemima, original complete	1/3 c	160	1.5	Na	0	1	6	0	15	0	+
Aunt Jemima, whole wheat	1/4 c	120	0.5	Na	0	3	4	0	6	0	+
Hungry Jack, buttermilk	1/5 c	150	1.5	Na	0	<1	5	0	15	0	0
Hungry Jack, extra light & fluffy	1/5 c	150	1.5	Na	0	<1	4	0	15	0	0
Hungry Jack, original	1/5 c	150	1.5	Na	0	<1	7	0	0	0	0
PANCAKE/WAFFLE (frozen)											
Aunt Jemima mini pancakes, strawberry	13	240	4	Na	1	1	6	0	10	0	+
Eggo, buttermilk pancakes	3	280	9	Na	1.5	1	11	0	4	0	+
Eggo, buttermilk waffles	2	180	6	Na	2	1	2	0	10	0	+
Eggo, chocolate chip waffles	2	210	7	Na	2.5	1	9	0	10	0	+
Eggo, Choco-'Nilla Flip-Flop waffles	2	190	7	Na	2	<1	7	0	10	0	+
Eggo, Special K waffles	2	190	1	0	0	1	5	0	15	0	‡
Pillsbury											
Blueberry pancakes	3	230	3.5	Na	0.5	2	14	Na	10	0	+
Buttermilk pancakes	3	240	4	Na	2	2	13	Na	10	0	+
Mini buttermilk pancakes	11	250	7	Na	3	<1	11	Na	8	0	+
Original pancakes	3	250	4	Na	2	2	14	Na	10	0	+
Waffles, blueberry	2	180	5	Na	3	1	6	Na	0	0	+
Waffles, buttermilk	2	170	5	3	3	1	4	Na	0	0	+
Waffles, homestyle	2	170	5	3	Na	1	4	Na	0	0	+
PANCAKE SYRUP											
Aunt Jemima, butter lite	1/4 c	100	0	0	0	1	25	0	0	0	0
Aunt Jemima, butter rich	1/4 c	210	0	0	0	0	29	0	0	0	0

Food	Portion Size	Calories	Total Fat (g)	Good Fats (g)	Bad Fats (g)	Fiber (g)	Sugars (mg)	Beta-carotene (mcg)	Calcium (%DV)	Vit. C (%DV)	B vit. (B_6,+,++)
Aunt Jemima, lite	¼ c	100	0	0	0	1	25	0	0	0	0
Aunt Jemima, original	¼ c	210	0	0	0	1	32	0	0	0	0
PAPAYA											
Fresh, cubed	1 c	55	0	0	0	3	8	386	3	144	+
Nectar (Knudsen)	8 oz	140	0	0	0	0	31	Na	2	25	+
Nectar, creamed (Knudsen)	8 oz	40	0	0	0	2	8	Na	0	60	+
PARSNIPS, fresh, cooked, no salt	½ c	55	0	0	0	3	4	0	2	16	+
PASTA (bowls/boxed)											
Betty Crocker											
Bowl Appetit, cheddar, broccoli, pasta bowl	1	330	11	Na	6.5	2	7	0	10	0	+
Bowl Appetit, chicken pasta bowl	1	260	6	Na	3	2	3	0	2	0	+
Bowl Appetit, garlic parmesan bowl	1	320	9	Na	5.5	1	5	0	10	0	+
Bowl Appetit, pasta alfredo bowl	1	360	11	Na	7.5	1	10	0	15	0	+
Bowl Appetit, three-cheese rotini bowl	1	360	10	Na	6.5	0	12	0	15	0	+
Chicken Helper, four cheese, mix	2/3 c	160	5	0	3.5	1	3	Na	4	0	+
Suddenly Pasta Salad, Caesar, mix	½ c	170	1	0	0	1	4	Na	2	0	+
Suddenly Pasta Salad, classic, mix	2/3 c	180	1	0	0	2	5	Na	4	0	+
Suddenly Pasta Salad, ranch & bacon, mix	½ c	160	1.5	0	0	1	3	Na	2	0	+
Tuna Helper, cheesy pasta, mix	½ c	140	1	0	0	1	1	Na	0	0	+
Tuna Helper, creamy broccoli, mix	½ c	170	1	0	0	2	2	Na	0	0	+
Tuna Helper, creamy pasta, mix	½ c	140	1	0	0	1	1	Na	0	0	+
Tuna Helper, fettuccine alfredo, mix	¾ c	170	3	Na	2	1	2	Na	2	0	+

Food	Portion Size	Calories	Total Fat (g)	Good Fats (g)	Bad Fats (g)	Fiber (g)	Sugars (mg)	Beta-carotene (mcg)	Calcium (%DV)	Vit. C (%DV)	B vit. (0,+,++)
Canned											
Chef Boyardee Beefaroni	1 c	236	7	3	3.5	1	5	0	3	0	0
Chef Boyardee mini beef ravioli meat sauce	1 c	240	8	3	3.5	2.5	5	0	3	0	0
Chef Boyardee beef ravioli, meat/tomato	1 c	224	6.5	3	3	1	5	0	3	0	0
Chef Boyardee spaghetti w/meatballs	1 c	257	10	4	4.5	3.5	7.5	Na	3	0	+
SpaghettiOs	1 c	180	1	Na	05	3	13	Na	2	0	+
SpaghettiOs, A to Z w/meatballs	1 c	260	9	Na	4	3	12	Na	15	10	+
SpaghettiOs, A to Z, w/sliced franks	1 c	230	10	Na	5	5	9	Na	15	10	+
SpaghettiOs, w/meatballs	1 c	240	8	Na	3.5	4	10	Na	15	10	+
SpaghettiOs plus calcium	1 c	170	1	Na	0.5	3	13	Na	30	10	+
Dry											
Corn, angel hair (Westbrae)	2 oz	210	1.5	0	0	0	0	0	0	0	0
Durum wheat, various brands	2 oz	210	1	0	0	1	1	0	1	0	+
Kamut, organic (Eden Foods)	2 oz	210	1.5	0.5	0.5	6	2	Na	2	2	+
Rye, organic (Eden Foods)	2 oz	200	0	0	0	8	1	Na	2	2	+
Spinach spaghetti (Westbrae)	2 oz	180	2	0	0	8	1	Na	2	0	+
Spelt ziti (Eden Foods)	2 oz	210	2	Na	0	5	1	Na	0	0	+
Whole wheat lasagna (Westbrae)	2 oz	180	1.5	Na	0	7	1	Na	0	0	+
Whole wheat spaghetti (Westbrae)	2 oz	200	1.5	Na	0	9	1	Na	0	0	+
Refrigerated											
Angel hair pasta	1 c	230	2.5	Na	1	2	1	4	2	0	Na
Linguine	1¼ c	240	2.5	Na	1	2	1	Na	2	0	Na
Ravioli, classic beef	1¼ c	350	10	Na	3	3	4	Na	6	0	Na
Ravioli, four cheese	1⅓ c	330	10	Na	6	3	3	Na	15	0	Na

Food	Portion Size	Calories	Total Fat (g)	Good Fats (g)	Bad Fats (g)	Fiber (g)	Sugars (mg)	Beta-carotene (mcg)	Calcium (%DV)	Vit. C (%DV)	B vit. (0,+,++)
Tortelloni, cheese & roasted garlic	1 c	270	8	Na	4	2	3	Na	15	0	Na
Tortelloni, mozzarella & pepperoni	1 c	330	10	Na	4.5	3	3	Na	15	0	Na
Tortellini, spinach cheese	1 c	320	7	Na	3.5	3	4	Na	20	0	Na
Tortellini, sweet Italian sausage	1 c	330	10	Na	3	3	6	Na	4	0	Na
Tortellini, three cheese	1 c	330	7	Na	3.5	3	4	Na	15	0	Na
PASTA SAUCE											
Buitoni											
Alfredo	½ c	130	11	Na	7	0	2	Na	10	0	0
Light Alfredo	½ c	90	6	Na	3.5	0	1	Na	10	0	0
Marinara	½ c	70	3	Na	0.5	2	7	Na	6	2	0
Pesto w/basil	¼ c	300	28	Na	5	2	4	Na	15	6	0
Tomato herb parmesan	½ c	130	8	Na	2.5	2	7	Na	10	2	0
Classico											
Alfredo	¼ c	120	11	Na	5	0	1	Na	4	0	0
Basil pesto	¼ c	230	21	Na	3	1	2	Na	6	0	0
Florentine spinach & cheese	½ c	80	5	Na	1	2	5	Na	6	40	0
Italian sausage w/pepper & onion	½ c	90	2	Na	1	2	8	Na	6	10	0
Roasted garlic	½ c	60	1	Na	0	2	8	Na	6	8	0
Tomato & basil	½ c	60	1	Na	0	2	6	Na	6	10	0
Del Monte											
Italian herb chunky	½ c	60	1	Na	0	<1	8	Na	4	4	0
Spaghetti sauce w/four cheeses	½ c	70	1.5	Na	0	3	10	Na	4	15	0
Spaghetti sauce w/meat	½ c	60	1	Na	0	3	9	Na	4	15	0
Spaghetti sauce w/mushrooms	½ c	60	0.5	0	0	2	9	Na	4	15	0

Food	Portion Size	Calories	Total Fat (g)	Good Fats (g)	Bad Fats (g)	Fiber (g)	Sugars (mg)	Beta-carotene (mcg)	Calcium (%DV)	Vit. C (%DV)	B vit. (0,+,++)
Eden Foods											
Pizza pasta sauce, organic	½ c	65	2.5	Na	0	5	4	Na	4	20	0
Spaghetti sauce, organic	½ c	80	2.5	Na	0	3	6	Na	8	20	0
Hunts											
Four cheese	½ c	50	1	0	0	3	7	Na	4	15	0
Meat	½ c	60	1	0	0	0	7	Na	2	15	0
Mushroom	½ c	50	1	0	0	3	7	Na	2	15	0
Muir Glen Organic											
Fire roasted tomato	½ c	70	2	Na	0	2	3	Na	4	35	0
Four cheese	½ c	80	2.5	Na	1	2	3	Na	6	15	0
Garden vegetable	½ c	60	1	Na	0	2	4	Na	2	15	0
Mushroom marinara	½ c	50	0	0	0	2	4	Na	2	10	0
Tomato basil	½ c	60	1	Na	0	2	4	Na	2	10	0
Newman's Own											
Bombolina	½ c	90	4.5	Na	0.5	<1	12	Na	2	0	0
Five cheese	½ c	80	3	Na	1.5	<1	0	Na	0	0	0
Italian sausage & pepper	½ c	90	4	Na	1	<1	9	Na	4	0	0
Marinara	½ c	70	2	Na	0	<1	11	Na	4	0	0
Pesto & tomato	½ c	80	4	Na	0.5	<1	9	Na	8	0	0
Prego											
Basil, tomato & garlic	½ c	90	2	Na	0.5	3	11	Na	2	2	0
Fresh mushroom	½ c	110	3.5	Na	1	3	11	Na	2	4	0
Italian sausage & garlic	½ c	120	5	Na	1.5	3	10	Na	2	2	0
Roasted garlic parmesan	½ c	100	1	0	0.5	3	13	Na	4	2	0

Food	Portion Size	Calories	Total Fat (g)	Good Fats (g)	Bad Fats (g)	Fiber (g)	Sugars (mg)	Beta-carotene (mcg)	Calcium (%DV)	Vit. C (%DV)	B vit. (0,+,++)
PASTRAMI											
Beef, 98% fat free	2 oz	54	1	0	0	0	0	0	0	32	+
Carl Buddig, beef, chopped, pressed	2 oz	80	4	0	2	0	0	0	0	0	0
Turkey	1 oz	67	2	1	1	0	2	1	0	4	0
PASTRY—Toaster											
Kellogg's Pop Tarts											
Apple cinnamon	1	210	6	3	2	<1	17	Na	0	0	+
Blueberry	1	210	6	3	2	<1	16	Na	0	0	+
Chocolate chip cookie dough	1	200	6	Na	2	<1	18	Na	0	0	+
French toast	1	220	8	Na	2.5	<1	15	Na	0	0	+
Frosted cherry	1	200	5	3	1.5	4	17	Na	0	0	+
Frosted chocolate fudge	1	200	5	2.5	1.5	<1	20	Na	2	0	+
Frosted cookies & crème	1	200	5	Na	2	<1	19	Na	2	0	+
Frosted raspberry	1	210	5	3	1.5	<1	19	Na	0	0	+
Low-fat frosted brown sugar cinnamon	1	190	3	1.5	1	<1	19	Na	0	0	+
Low-fat frosted strawberry	1	190	3	1.5	1	<1	20	Na	0	0	+
Pillsbury Toaster Strudel											
Apple	1	190	9	Na	4.5	<1	9	Na	0	0	Na
Blueberry	1	190	9	Na	4.5	<1	9	Na	0	0	Na
Chocolate fudge	1	210	10	Na	5.5	<1	9	Na	0	0	Na
Cream cheese & raspberry	1	200	10	Na	5	<1	8	Na	0	0	Na
Strawberry	1	190	9	Na	4.5	<1	9	Na	0	0	Na
Wild berry	1	190	9	Na	4.5	<1	9	Na	0	0	Na

Food	Portion Size	Calories	Total Fat (g)	Good Fats (g)	Bad Fats (g)	Fiber (g)	Sugars (mg)	Beta-carotene (mcg)	Calcium (%DV)	Vit. C (%DV)	B vit. (0,+,++)
PEACHES, fresh raw, 2.5" diameter	1	38	0	0	0	1	8	158	0	10	0
Canned											
Del Monte, carb clever, sliced	½ c	30	0	0	0	1	6	Na	0	80	0
Del Monte, freestone slices	½ c	100	0	0	0	1	23	Na	0	2	0
Del Monte fruit naturals, chunks	½ c	70	0	0	0	<1	16	Na	0	100	0
Del Monte harvest spice, sliced	½ c	80	0	0	0	<1	20	Na	0	6	0
S&W, halves	½ c	70	0	0	0	1	16	Na	0	2	0
S&W, natural style	½ c	80	0	0	0	1	18	Na	0	2	0
S&W snow peaches	½ c	80	0	0	0	1	19	Na	0	100	0
Dried, sulfured, halves	1 c	382	2	0.5	0	13	67	1718	4	12	+
Frozen, Cascadian Farm, sliced, organic	1 c	50	0	0	0	2	12	Na	0	210	0
Juice, Nectar											
Knudsen	8 oz	130	0	0	0	0	28	Na	2	0	Na
Santa Cruz, organic	8 oz	120	0	0	0	0	29	Na	0	0	0
PEANUT BUTTER											
Jif, creamy	2 tbs	190	16	7.5*	3	2	3	0	0	0	0
Jif, creamy & honey	2 tbs	190	15	7.5	2.5	2	7	0	0	0	0
Jif, reduced fat	2 tbs	190	12	Na	2.5	1	4	0	2	0	0
Maranatha organic, creamy & roasted	2 tbs	190	16	Na	2	3	3	0	2	0	0
Maranatha organic, crunchy	2 tbs	190	16	Na	2	3	1	0	2	0	0
Skippy, honey roasted creamy	2 tbs	190	17	Na	3.5	2	3	0	0	0	0
Skippy, reduced fat, creamy	2 tbs	190	12	Na	2.5	2	5	0	0	0	0
Skippy, regular creamy	2 tbs	190	17	Na	3.5	2	3	0	0	0	0
Skippy, super chunk	2 tbs	190	17	Na	3.5	2	3	0	0	0	0

Food	Portion Size	Calories	Total Fat (g)	Good Fats (g)	Bad Fats (g)	Fiber (g)	Sugars (mg)	Beta-carotene (mcg)	Calcium (%DV)	Vit. C (%DV)	B vit. (0,+,++)
Smart Balance omega, creamy	2 tbs	200	17	12	2.5	2	2	0	0	0	+
Smuckers natural, creamy or chunky	2 tbs	210	16	Na	2.5	2	1	0	0	0	0
Smuckers natural, reduced fat creamy	2 tbs	200	12	Na	2	2	2	0	0	0	0
PEANUTS											
Dry roasted, w/salt	1 oz	165	14	7	2	2	1	0	2	0	+
Oil roasted, w/salt	1 oz	169	15	7	2	2	1	0	1	0	+
Planters, honey roasted	1 oz	160	13	Na	1.5	2	4	0	0	0	+
PEARS, fresh, raw, medium	1	96	0	0	0	5	16	21	1	11	0
Canned/jarred											
Del Monte, Bartlett, cinnamon halves	1/2 c	80	0	0	0	1	19	0	0	2	0
Del Monte, Bartlett, halves	1/2 c	60	0	0	0	1	14	0	0	4	0
Del Monte, Bartlett, Orchard Select	1/2 c	80	0	0	0	2	19	0	0	100	0
S&W, Bartlett, halves, light syrup	1/2 c	80	0	0	0	2	17	0	0	2	0
S&W, Bartlett, slices, natural style	1/2 c	80	0	0	0	2	17	0	0	2	0
Nectar, Santa Cruz, organic	8 oz	120	0	0	0	0	25	Na	4	4	0
PEAS, fresh, boiled, no salt	1 c	134	0	0	0	0	0	0	2	11	0
Canned											
Del Monte, peas & carrots	1/2 c	60	0	0	0	2	4	0	2	6	0
Del Monte, sweet peas	1/2 c	60	0	0	0	4	6	0	2	15	0
Del Monte, very young small sweet	1/2 c	60	0	0	0	4	5	0	0	15	0
Green Giant, LeSueur early peas	2/3 c	60	0.5	0	0	3	4	0	2	10	0
Frozen											
Green Giant, baby sweet peas & butter	3/4 c	80	1.5	0	1	4	5	0	2	20	0
Green Giant, select early June peas	2/3 c	60	0.5	0	0	4	3	0	2	20	0

Food	Portion Size	Calories	Total Fat (g)	Good Fats (g)	Bad Fats (g)	Fiber (g)	Sugars (mg)	Beta-carotene (mcg)	Calcium (%DV)	Vit. C (%DV)	B vit. (0,+,++)
PECANS, raw, halves	1 oz	193	20	11.5	2	3	2	8	1	0	0
Planters, chips	2 oz	390	40	23*	3	7	2	0	4	2	+
PEPPERS											
Fresh, raw, green, chopped	1 c	30	0	0	0	3	4	310	1	199	0
Fresh, raw, red, chopped	1 c	39	0	0	0	3	6	2419	1	471	0
Fresh, raw, yellow, chopped, large 3"	1	50	0	0	0	2	0	233	2	568	+
PEPPERONI											
Bridgford, original	1 oz	130	12	Na	1	0	0	0	0	2	Na
Smart Deli (soy), slices	13 slices	40	0	0	0	1	<1	0	4	0	Na
PICKLES											
Cascadian Farms, baby dills	1½ pc	5	0	0	0	0	0	0	0	0	0
Cascadian Farms, bread & butter chips	5 slices	30	0	0	0	0	2	0	0	0	0
Claussen bread 'n butter sandwich slices	1 oz	5	0	0	0	0	0	0	0	0	0
Claussen, kosher dill halves or spears	1 oz	5	0	0	0	0	0	0	0	0	0
Claussen sweet gerkins	1 oz	30	0	0	0	0	6	0	0	2	0
Del Monte, sweet, midget	1 oz	40	0	0	0	<1	10	0	0	0	0
Del Monte, sweet, whole	1 oz	40	0	0	0	<1	10	0	0	0	0
PIES, frozen											
Edward's chocolate butter pecan	1 pc	560	32	Na	14	2	36	0	8	0	0
Edward's chocolate cream	⅛ pie	450	27	Na	18	1	33	0	8	0	0
Edward's Georgia pecan	⅛ pie	490	22	Na	16.5	1	26	0	0	0	0
Edward's key lime	⅛ pie	450	26	Na	8	0	47	0	20	0	0
Edward's Oreo cream	⅛ pie	480	30	Na	20.5	2	35	0	8	0	0

Food	Portion Size	Calories	Total Fat (g)	Good Fats (g)	Bad Fats (g)	Fiber (g)	Sugars (mg)	Beta-carotene (mcg)	Calcium (%DV)	Vit. C (%DV)	B vit. (0,+,++)
Edward's turtle	1/8 pie	390	22	Na	13.5	1	32	0	6	0	0
Sara Lee, apple	1/8 pie	340	15	Na	7	1	26	0	0	2	0
Sara Lee, blueberry	1/8 pie	360	15	Na	7	2	26	0	2	4	0
Sara Lee, cherry	1/8 pie	330	15	Na	3.5	2	27	0	2	2	0
Sara Lee, Dutch apple	1/8 pie	350	15	Na	6	2	30	0	2	2	0
Sara Lee, mince	1/8 pie	390	17	Na	4	3	30	0	2	4	0
Sara Lee, peach deep dish	1/10 pie	370	21	Na	9.5	2	18	0	0	0	0
Sara Lee, pumpkin homestyle	1/8 pie	260	11	Na	2.5	2	18	0	6	0	0
Sara Lee, tropical coconut cream	1/8 pie	450	27	Na	18	1	29	0	4	0	0
PIE CRUST											
Pet-Ritz, deep dish	1/8 crust	90	5	Na	2	0	1	0	0	0	0
Pet-Ritz, deep dish, all vegetable	1/8 crust	90	5	Na	2.5	0	1	0	0	0	0
Pet-Ritz, regular	1/8 crust	80	4	Na	1.5	0	1	0	0	0	0
PIE FILLING											
Lucky Leaf											
Apple	1/3 c	90	0	0	0	2	17	Na	0	0	0
Apricot	1/3 c	90	0	0	0	0	13	Na	0	25	0
Blueberry, premium	1/3 c	100	0	0	0	1	17	Na	0	0	0
Coconut crème	1/3 c	110	2	0	0	3	12	Na	0	0	0
Lemon cream	1/3 c	130	1	0	0	0	15	Na	0	2	0
Pineapple	1/3 c	100	0	0	0	1	13	Na	0	2	0
Raisin	1/3 c	90	0	0	0	1	15	Na	0	2	0
Strawberry, premium	1/2 c	100	0	0	0	1	16	Na	0	6	0

Food	Portion Size	Calories	Total Fat (g)	Good Fats (g)	Bad Fats (g)	Fiber (g)	Sugars (mg)	Beta-carotene (mcg)	Calcium (%DV)	Vit. C (%DV)	B vit. (0,+,++)
PIEROGIES											
Mrs. T, American cheese	3	210	6	Na	3	1	1	Na	8	8	0
Mrs. T, broccoli & cheddar	3	200	4.5	Na	2	2	2	Na	4	20	0
Mrs. T, four cheese	3	230	7	Na	1.5	1	2	Na	4	15	0
Mrs. T, sour cream & chives	3	210	5	Na	2.5	1	2	Na	4	15	0
PINEAPPLE, fresh, diced	1 c	74	0	0	0	2	14	53	2	93	0
Del Monte, chunks in own juice	½ c	70	0	0	0	1	15	Na	0	20	0
Del Monte, Fruit Naturals	½ c	70	0	0	0	<1	15	10*	0	100	0
Dole, fruit bowl	4 oz	60	0	0	0	1	14	Na	0	40	0
Dole, fruit bowl in lime gel	4.3 oz	90	0	0	0	0	22	Na	0	40	0
Dole, slices in 100% juice	2 slices	60	0	0	0	1	13	Na	0	25	0
Dole, tidbits in 100% juice	½ c	60	0	0	0	1	13	Na	0	25	0
PINEAPPLE JUICE/BEVERAGE											
Dole, 100%	8 oz	120	0	0	0	0	29	Na	2	100	0
Dole, pineapple orange, 100%	6 oz	100	0	0	0	0	18	Na	2	100	0
Knudsen, nectar	8 oz	140	0	0	0	0	26	Na	2	15	0
Knudsen, pineapple coconut	8 oz	130	1	Na	0.5	0	27	Na	4	0	0
Santa Cruz, orange pineapple	8 oz	130	0	0	0	0	29	Na	0	15	0
Santa Cruz, pineapple coconut	8 oz	130	0.5	0	0.5	0	28	Na	2	0	0
PISTACHIOS, dry roasted (Planters)	1 oz	170	14	7	2	3	2	44	3	1	+
PIZZA (frozen) (Also see Fast Food)											
Amy's Kitchen											
Cheese	⅓ pie	310	12	Na	4	2	4	Na	20	6	0
Mediterranean w/cornmeal crust	⅓ pie	360	15	Na	4.5	3	2	Na	20	10	0

183

Food	Portion Size	Calories	Total Fat (g)	Good Fats (g)	Bad Fats (g)	Fiber (g)	Sugars (mg)	Beta-carotene (mcg)	Calcium (%DV)	Vit. C (%DV)	B vit. (0,+,++)
Pesto	1/3 pie	310	12	Na	3.5	2	3	Na	15	15	0
Rice crust, cheese	1/3 pie	300	14	Na	4	2	5	Na	20	8	0
Roasted vegetable	1/3 pie	270	9	Na	1.5	2	5	Na	2	20	0
Soy cheese	1/3 pie	290	11	Na	1	2	3	Na	2	4	0
Three cheese w/cornmeal crust	1/3 pie	370	19	Na	4	2	6	Na	10	10	0
DiGiorno											
Cheese stuffed crust, 3 meat	1/6 pie	340	16	Na	7.5	2	5	Na	20	0	0
Cheese stuffed crust, pepperoni	1/5 pie	370	16	Na	8.5	3	6	Na	25	0	0
Cheese stuffed crust, 4 cheese	1/5 pie	360	15	Na	8.5	3	6	Na	30	0	0
Deep dish, 3 meat	1/6 pie	340	18	Na	8.5	2	5	Na	20	0	0
Deep dish, supreme	1/6 pie	320	15	Na	7.5	2	5	Na	15	0	0
Microwave rising crust, pepperoni	1/2 pie	390	18	Na	8.5	3	7	Na	15	0	0
Microwave rising crust, supreme	1/2 pie	400	18	Na	8.5	4	7	Na	15	6	0
Thin crispy crust, harvest wheat supreme	1/5 pie	250	8	Na	3.5	4	5	Na	15	6	Na
Thin crispy crust, harvest wheat pepperoni	1/5 pie	270	9	Na	4	4	5	Na	25	2	0
Thin crispy crust, supreme	1/5 pie	300	12	Na	5	3	8	Na	15	6	0
Jeno's Crisp 'n Tasty											
Canadian bacon	1 pie	420	18	Na	8	2	6	Na	15	0	0
Cheese	1 pie	440	21	Na	10	2	5	Na	30	0	0
Combination	1 pie	490	25	12*	10.5	2	5	Na	15	0	0
Hamburger	1 pie	480	22	Na	9.5	2	5	Na	15	0	0
Pepperoni	1 pie	490	26	14*	11	2	5	Na	15	0	0
Sausage	1 pie	480	24	Na	10.5	2	5	Na	15	0	0

Food	Portion Size	Calories	Total Fat (g)	Good Fats (g)	Bad Fats (g)	Fiber (g)	Sugars (mg)	Beta-carotene (mcg)	Calcium (%DV)	Vit. C (%DV)	B vit. (0,+,++)
Supreme	1 pie	490	25	Na	10.5	2	5	Na	15	0	0
Three meat	1 pie	480	24	Na	10.5	2	5	Na	15	0	0
Lean Cuisine											
Cheese French bread	1 pkg	320	7	0.5	4	4	8	Na	25	15	0
Delux French bread	1 pkg	310	9	0.5	3.5	3	7	Na	15	25	0
Pepperoni French bread	1 pkg	290	8	0.5	3	3	7	Na	15	10	0
Tombstone											
Brickoven pepperoni	¼ pie	310	16	Na	7	2	4	Na	20	4	0
Brickoven pepperoni & sausage	¼ pie	320	16	Na	7	3	4	Na	20	2	0
Brickoven, supreme	¼ pie	320	16	Na	7	3	4	Na	20	4	0
Harvest wheat thin crust, cheese	⅓ pie	300	10	Na	5	4	5	Na	30	4	0
Harvest wheat thin crust, supreme	¼ pie	260	10	Na	4.5	3	4	Na	20	4	0
Light veggie	⅕ pie	230	6	Na	2	4	15	Na	20	4	0
Original, sausage & mushroom	⅕ pie	306	15	4.5	5	0	0	145	20	0	0
Original, extra cheese	¼ pie	350	15	Na	8.5	4	5	Na	35	0	0
Original, supreme	⅕ pie	300	14	Na	6	3	5	Na	20	0	0
Original, 4 meat	⅕ pie	310	14	Na	6	3	4	Na	20	0	0
Totino's Party Pizza											
Canadian bacon	½ pie	320	15	Na	7	1	4	Na	15	0	0
Cheese	½ pie	320	15	Na	7	1	4	Na	20	0	0
Combination	½ pie	380	21	10*	9	1	7	Na	15	0	0
Hamburger	½ pie	360	19	Na	9	1	7	Na	15	0	0
Mexican	½ pie	370	19	Na	9	2	3	Na	15	0	0
Mini meatball	½ pie	350	18	Na	8	1	3	Na	15	0	0

Food	Portion Size	Calories	Total Fat (g)	Good Fats (g)	Bad Fats (g)	Fiber (g)	Sugars (mg)	Beta-carotene (mcg)	Calcium (%DV)	Vit. C (%DV)	B vit. (0,+,++)
Pepperoni	½ pie	360	20	10*	9	3	4	Na	15	0	0
Sausage	½ pie	360	19	Na	8	1	4	Na	15	0	0
Supreme	½ pie	360	19	Na	8.5	1	4	Na	15	0	0
Three cheese	½ pie	330	16	Na	7.5	1	4	Na	25	0	0
Three meat	½ pie	350	18	Na	8	1	3	Na	15	0	0
PIZZA SNACKS											
Totino's pizza rolls, cheese	6 rolls	190	6	3*	3	1	4	Na	0	0	0
Totino's pizza rolls, cheesy taco	6 rolls	210	10	5*	5	1	2	Na	8	0	0
Totino's pizza rolls, combination	6 rolls	220	11	5*	4.5	1	2	Na	4	0	0
Totino's pizza rolls, pepperoni	6 rolls	210	10	5*	4	1	3	Na	4	0	0
Totino's pizza rolls, sausage	6 rolls	210	10	5*	4	1	3	Na	4	0	0
Totino's pizza rolls, supreme	6 rolls	210	9	4*	3.5	2	3	Na	4	0	0
Totino's pizza rolls, three meat	6 rolls	210	9	4*	4	1	3	Na	4	0	0
PLANTAIN, raw	1 c	181	1	0	0	3	22	676	0	45	+
PLUMS, raw, 2⅛" diameter	1	30	0	0	0	1	7	125	0	10	0
Canned, purple, light syrup	1 c	159	0	0	0	2	39	320	2	1	0
POMEGRANATE											
Fresh fruit, 3⅜"	1	104	0	0	0	0	26	61	0	15	0
Knudsen, Just Pomegranate	8 oz	150	0	0	0	0	36	Na	0	2	0
Knudsen, Vita Pomegranate	8 oz	130	0	0	0	0	28	Na	15	100	0
POM, 100%	8 oz	160	0	0	0	0	34	Na	0	0	0
POPCORN											
Air-popped, plain, no salt	1 c	31	0	0	0	1	0	0	0	0	0
Jolly Time, microwave, healthy pop, kernels	2 tbs	90	2	0	0	9	0	0	0	0	0

Food	Portion Size	Calories	Total Fat (g)	Good Fats (g)	Bad Fats (g)	Fiber (g)	Sugars (mg)	Beta-carotene (mcg)	Calcium (%DV)	Vit. C (%DV)	B vit. (0,+,++)
Jolly Time, microwave, sassy salsa, kernels	2 tbs	160	11	Na	7	3	0	0	0	0	0
Jolly Time, microwave, mallow magic, kernels	2 tbs	180	13	Na	2.5	3	5	0	0	0	0
Wise, bagged, butter flavored	1 oz	150	10	Na	2	3	0	0	0	0	0
Wise, bagged, hot cheese	1 oz	150	10	Na	2	2	3	Na	2	0	0
Wise, bagged, lite butter flavored	1 oz	140	5	Na	1	3	0	Na	0	0	0
Wise, bagged, white cheddar	1 oz	150	10	Na	2.5	2	2	Na	4	0	0
PORK											
Fresh, center loin chops, lean & fat, broiled	3 oz	204	11	5	4	0	0	0	2	0	+
Fresh, center rib chops, lean & fat, broiled	3 oz	224	13	6	5	0	0	0	2	0	+
Fresh, center rib roast, lean, roasted	3 oz	182	9	4	3	0	0	0	2	0	+
Fresh, loin blade chops, lean & fat, broiled	3 oz	272	21	9	8	0	0	0	2	0	+
Fresh, spare ribs, braised, lean & fat	3 oz	337	26	11.5	9	0	0	0	3	0	+
Fresh, tenderloin, lean, roasted	3 oz	139	4	1.5	1	0	0	0	0	0	+
Fresh, tenderloin, lean & fat, roasted	3 oz	147	5	2	2	0	0	0	0	2	+
Hormel, Always Tender, boneless loin	4 oz	162	8	4	3	0	0	0	0	2	0
Hormel, Always Tender, center chops	4 oz	187	11	5	4	0	0	0	0	2	0
Hormel, Always Tender, fillets, lemon-garlic	4 oz	132	5	2	2	0	0	0	1	3	0
Hormel, Always Tender, tenderloin, peppercorn	4 oz	123	4	1.5	1	0	0	0	1	3	0
PORK RINDS											
Wise hot & spicy, BBQ	0.625 oz	90	5	5	1	0	0	0	0	2	0
Wise, original	0.625 oz	90	6	Na	2	1.5	0	0	0	0	0
Wise, sweet & mild BBQ	0.625 oz	90	6	Na	2	0	1	0	0	0	0

POTATOES

Food	Portion Size	Calories	Total Fat (g)	Good Fats (g)	Bad Fats (g)	Fiber (g)	Sugars (mg)	Beta-carotene (mcg)	Calcium (%DV)	Vit. C (%DV)	B vit. (0,+,++)
Baked, skin & flesh, 2¼–3¼" dia.	1	161	0	0	0	4	2	10	2	27	+
Boiled, skin & flesh, 2½" dia.	1	118	0	0	0	3	1	3	0	29	0
Canned											
Del Monte, au gratin	½ c	80	2.5	Na	1	1	1	0	4	10	0
Del Monte, w/green beans & ham flavor	½ c	30	0	0	0	<1	1	0	2	8	0
Del Monte, new potatoes, sliced	⅔ c	60	0	0	0	2	0	0	2	15	0
Frozen											
Birds Eye, roasted potatoes & broccoli	⅔ c	100	4	Na	2	1	0	0	4	25	0
Cascadian Farm, country style	¾ c	50	0	0	0	1	0	0	0	8	0
Cascadian Farm, crinkle cut French fries	18 pcs	130	4	Na	1	2	1	0	0	8	0
Cascadian Farm, hash browns	1 c	60	0	0	0	1	0	0	0	8	0
Cascadian Farm, spud puppies	10 pcs	160	7	Na	2	2	1	0	0	6	0
Cascadian Farm, wedge cut	8 pcs	110	3	Na	1	2	1	0	0	8	0
McCain, mash bites	3 oz	170	7	Na	0.5	2	1	0	2	0	0
McCain, Roasters All-American	3 oz	120	3	Na	0	2	<1	0	0	6	0
McCain, Roasters, French onion	3 oz	110	3	Na	0	2	<1	0	0	8	0
McCain, Roasters, grilled garlic & onion	3 oz	120	3	Na	0	2	1	0	0	8	0
McCain, seasoned beer-battered wedges	3 oz	140	7	Na	4	2	<1	0	0	8	0
McCain seasoned spirals	3 oz	140	7	Na	0.5	2	<1	0	2	4	0
McCain seasoned wedges w/skin	3 oz	120	5	Na	0	2	<1	0	0	4	0
McCain shoestring	45 pcs	140	5	Na	0.5	2	0	0	0	6	0
McCain steak fries	8 pcs	120	4	Na	0	2	0	0	0	6	0
McCain Tasti Tater shaped	8 pcs	160	7	Na	0.5	3	<1	0	0	4	0

Food	Portion Size	Calories	Total Fat (g)	Good Fats (g)	Bad Fats (g)	Fiber (g)	Sugars (mg)	Beta-carotene (mcg)	Calcium (%DV)	Vit. C (%DV)	B vit. (0,+,++)
Mixes/Boxed—Betty Crocker											
Au gratin	½ c	100	1.5	Na	1	1	2	15*	2	0	0
Butter & herb mash	½ c	90	1	Na	1	1	1	0	2	0	0
Cheddar & bacon	⅔ c	100	1.5	Na	1	1	1	Na	2	0	0
Delux cheesy cheddar	⅔ c	130	4.5	Na	2.5	1	2	Na	6	0	0
Delux creamy scallop	½ c	140	4.5	Na	2.5	1	2	Na	4	0	0
Hash browns, Seasoned Skillets	½ c	90	0.5	0	0	2	0	Na	0	0	0
Homestyle cheesey scalloped	⅔ c	100	1.5	0	1	2	1	Na	0	0	0
Homestyle creamy butter mash	½ c	90	1	0	0	1	1	Na	0	0	0
Julienne	⅓ c	90	1	0	0	1	2	Na	2	0	0
Roasted garlic scalloped	⅔ c	90	1.5	0	1	1	1	Na	2	0	0
Specialty scalloped	½ c	90	1	0	1	1	1	Na	2	0	0
Specialty sour cream & chives scalloped	⅔ c	100	1	0	0.5	1	1	Na	2	0	0
Mixes/Boxed—Idahoan											
Hash browns, mix	⅓ c	90	0.5	0	0	1	0	Na	2	2	0
Mashed 4 cheese, mix	¼ c	100	2.5	Na	1	1	2	Na	4	15	0
Mashed herb & butter, mix	¼ c	110	2.5	Na	1	1	2	Na	2	15	0
Mashed homestyle, mix	¼ c	110	2.5	Na	1	1	2	Na	2	10	0
Mashed, original, mix	⅓ c	80	0	0	0	2	0	Na	0	6	0
POTATO CHIPS											
Herrs											
Bacon & horseradish	1 oz	160	10	Na	1.5	1	0	0	0	0	0
BBQ	1 oz	150	10	Na	3	1	4	0	0	0	0
Ketchup	1 oz	150	10	Na	2.5	1	3	0	0	0	0

189

Food	Portion Size	Calories	Total Fat (g)	Good Fats (g)	Bad Fats (g)	Fiber (g)	Sugars (mg)	Beta-carotene (mcg)	Calcium (%DV)	Vit. C (%DV)	B vit. (0,+,++)
Kettle cooked, jalapeno	1 oz	160	10	Na	2.5	1	3	0	0	0	0
Sour cream & onion	1 oz	150	10	Na	3	1	3	0	0	0	0
Lay's											
Baked, cheddar & sour cream	1 oz	120	3.5	Na	1	2	3	0	2	2	0
Baked, original crisps	1 oz	110	1.5	Na	0	2	2	0	4	2	0
Kettle cooked, jalapeno	1 oz	140	8	4.5	1	1	0	0	0	10	0
Kettle cooked, mesquite BBQ	1 oz	140	8	4.5	1	<1	1	0	0	10	0
Kettle cooked, original	1 oz	150	8	4.5	1	1	1	0	0	10	0
Natural thick cut country BBQ	1 oz	150	9	Na	1	1	1	0	2	10	0
Stax, cheddar flavored	1 oz	150	10	Na	2.5	1	1	0	2	2	0
Stax, Hidden Valley ranch	1 oz	150	9	Na	2.5	1	2	0	2	0	0
Stax, original	1 oz	160	10	Na	2.5	1	2	0	0	2	0
Stax, salt & vinegar	1 oz	150	9	Na	2.5	1	2	0	2	2	0
Wavy, au gratin	1 oz	150	10	6	1	1	<1	0	0	10	0
Wavy, hickory BBQ	1 oz	150	9	5.5	1	1	<1	0	0	8	0
Pringles											
Chili cheese	1 oz	160	10	Na	3	<1	1	0	0	6	0
Jalapeno	1 oz	150	10	Na	3	<1	1	0	0	6	0
Loaded baked potato	1 oz	150	10	Na	3	<1	1	Na	0	6	0
Pizza	1 oz	150	10	Na	3	<1	1	0	2	6	0
Original	1 oz	160	11	Na	3	<1	1	0	0	6	0
Ranch	1 oz	160	10	Na	3	<1	1	0	2	6	0
Sour cream & onion	1 oz	160	10	Na	3	<1	1	0	0	6	0

Food	Portion Size	Calories	Total Fat (g)	Good Fats (g)	Bad Fats (g)	Fiber (g)	Sugars (mg)	Beta-carotene (mcg)	Calcium (%DV)	Vit. C (%DV)	B vit. (0,+,++)
Wise											
BBQ flavored	1 oz	150	10	Na	3	1	4	0	0	10	0
Chipotle flavored	1 oz	150	10	Na	2	1	<1	0	0	10	0
Kettle cooked, jalapeno	1 oz	140	8	Na	2.5	1	0	0	0	10	0
Kettle cooked, natural	1 oz	150	9	Na	2.5	1	0	0	0	10	0
Original flat cut	1 oz	150	10	Na	3	1	0	0	0	10	0
PRETZELS											
Bachman											
Butter twists	1 oz	110	1	0	0	1	1	Na	0	0	0
Classic twist	1 oz	100	1	0	0	1	1	Na	0	0	0
Nutzels	1 oz	110	1	0	0	1	1	Na	0	0	0
Peanut butter pretzels	1 oz	160	8	Na	1.5	1	2	Na	0	0	0
Sourdough bites	1 oz	110	1	0	0	1	1	Na	0	0	0
Wheat & honey pretzelmack	1 oz	110	1	0	0	1	2	Na	0	0	0
Herr's											
Bite size hard	1 oz	100	0	0	0	2	2	Na	0	0	0
Chocolate covered rods	7/10 oz	90	2.5	Na	2	0	5	Na	2	0	0
Extra dark specials	1 oz	110	1	0	0	2	2	Na	2	0	0
Honey wheat	1 oz	110	2	Na	0	2	3	Na	2	0	0
Peanut butter filled	10 pcs	160	8	Na	1.5	1	2	Na	0	0	0
Specials	1½ oz	170	2	Na	0	2	0	Na	0	0	0
Rold Gold											
Cheddar tiny twists	1 oz	110	1	0	0	1	<1	Na	0	0	0
Classic rods	1 oz	110	1	0	0	1	1	Na	0	0	0

191

Food	Portion Size	Calories	Total Fat (g)	Good Fats (g)	Bad Fats (g)	Fiber (g)	Sugars (mg)	Beta-carotene (mcg)	Calcium (%DV)	Vit. C (%DV)	B vit. (0,+,++)
Fat-free tiny twists	1 oz	100	0	0	0	1	<1	Na	0	0	0
Hard sourdough	1 oz	100	0.5	0	0	1	<1	Na	0	0	0
Honey mustard tiny twists	1 oz	110	1	0	0	1	1	Na	0	0	0
Snyders of Hanover											
Butter snaps	1 oz	120	1	0	0	1	<1	Na	0	0	0
Honey wheat sticks	1 oz	120	2	Na	0	2	4	Na	0	0	0
Sourdough hard	1 oz	100	0	0	0	1	0	Na	0	0	0
12-grain sticks	1 oz	120	2	Na	0	3	3	Na	2	2	0
Superpretzel–Frozen											
Pretzelfils, mozzarella	2	130	3.5	Na	1.5	1	0	Na	8	0	0
Pretzelfils, pepperjack	2	130	3.5	Na	1.5	1	1	Na	6	0	0
Pretzelfils, pizza	2	130	2	0	2	1	1	Na	6	0	0
Soft pretzel, w/o added salt	1	160	1	0	0	1	1	Na	0	0	0
Soft pretzel bites w/o added salt	5 pcs	150	0.5	0	0	1	1	Na	0	0	0
Softstix	2	130	3	Na	1.5	1	1	Na	4	0	0
PRUNES/PRUNE BEVERAGE											
Knudsen, juice, organic	8 oz	170	0	0	0	3	27	Na	4	4	Na
Sunsweet bite size or whole prunes	1.5 oz	100	0	0	0	3	12	Na	2	0	0
Sunsweet ready to serve	2/3 c	150	0	0	0	3	24	Na	2	0	0
Sunsweet, juice w/ or w/o pulp	8 oz	180	0	0	0	3	18	Na	2	0	+
PUDDING											
Handi-Snacks, banana or vanilla	3.5 oz	90	1	0	0	0	15	Na	2	0	0
Handi-Snacks, chocolate	3.5 oz	100	1	0	1	1	17	Na	2	0	0
Handi-Snacks, chocolate, fat free	3.5 oz	90	0	0	0	0	16	Na	0	0	0

Food	Portion Size	Calories	Total Fat (g)	Good Fats (g)	Bad Fats (g)	Fiber (g)	Sugars (mg)	Beta-carotene (mcg)	Calcium (%DV)	Vit. C (%DV)	B vit. (0,+,++)
Handi-Snacks, double fudge, rocky road	3.5 oz	100	1	0	1	1	17	Na	2	0	0
Handi-Snacks, rice	3.5 oz	140	6	Na	1	0	11	Na	8	0	0
Jell-O											
Banana cream, cook & serve	½ c	80	0	0	0	0	15	Na	0	0	0
Banana cream, instant	½ c	90	0	0	0	0	18	Na	0	0	0
Butterscotch, instant	½ c	90	0	0	0	0	18	Na	0	0	0
Cheesecake, instant	½ c	100	0	0	0	0	20	Na	0	0	0
Chocolate, cook & serve	½ c	90	0	0	0	1	15	Na	0	0	0
Chocolate, cook & serve, sugar free	½ c	30	0	0	0	1	0	Na	0	0	0
Chocolate fudge, sugar & fat free	½ c	30	0	0	0	1	0	Na	0	0	0
Coconut cream, cook & serve	½ c	90	2.5	0	2.5	1	14	Na	2	0	0
Lemon, instant	½ c	90	0	0	0	0	19	Na	0	0	0
Mixed berry, Smoothie Snack	1 serv	100	2.5	Na	1.5	0	15	Na	2	0	0
Pistachio, instant	½ c	100	2.5	0	0	0	18	Na	0	0	0
Vanilla, cook & serve	½ c	80	0	0	0	0	16	Na	0	0	0
Uncle Ben's, cinnamon & raisin rice pudding	½ c	160	1	0	0	0	15	Na	2	0	0
PUMPKIN											
Fresh, cooked, no salt, mashed	1 c	49	0	0	0	3	2	5135	3	19	0
Seeds, kernels, roasted, no salt	1 oz	147	12	3.5	2	1	0	63	1	0	0
Seeds, whole, roasted, no salt	1 oz	126	5	1.5	1	0	0	0	1	0	0
PUNCH											
Hi-C Crazy Citrus, Orange Lavaburst	200 mL	100	0	0	0	0	25	0	0	100	0
Hi-C Boppin' Strawberry, Lemonade	200 mL	100	0	0	0	0	26	0	0	100	0

Food	Portion Size	Calories	Total Fat (g)	Good Fats (g)	Bad Fats (g)	Fiber (g)	Sugars (mg)	Beta-carotene (mcg)	Calcium (%DV)	Vit. C (%DV)	B vit. (0,+,++)
Hi-C Blast, Berry Blue	8 oz	120	0	0	0	0	31	Na	0	100	0
Hi-C Blast, Fruit Pow	1 bottle	180	0	0	0	0	45	Na	0	100	0
Hi-C Blast, orange, pouch	200 mL	100	0	0	0	0	25	Na	0	100	0
Kool-Aid mix, tropical punch	8 oz	60	0	0	0	0	16	0	0	10	0
Minute Maid, berry, citrus, grape, carton	8 oz	120	0	0	0	0	31	0	0	0	0
Minute Maid, tropical, carton	8 oz	110	0	0	0	0	29	Na	0	0	0
Tropicana fruit punch	8 oz	130	0	0	0	0	32	Na	2	100	+
QUINOA (Eden Foods)	1/4 c	180	3.5	0.5	0	11	2	0	2	0	0
RADISHES, raw, slices	1/2 c	9	0	0	0	1	1	2	0	14	0
RAISINS											
Dole	1/4 c	130	0	0	0	2	29	0	2	0	+
Sun-Maid, baking	1/4 c	110	0	0	0	2	25	0	2	0	+
Sun-Maid, chocolate covered	30 pcs	170	6	Na	4	1	25	0	4	0	+
Sun-Maid, chocolate yogurt	1/4 c	120	4	Na	3.5	1	19	0	4	0	+
Sun-Maid, golden or regular	1/4 c	130	0	0	0	2	29	0	2	2	+
Sun-Maid, vanilla yogurt	1/4 c	130	5	Na	4	1	19	0	4	2	+
RASPBERRIES, raw, red	1 c	64	1	0	0	28	5	15	3	53	0
Cascadian Farm, organic, frozen	1 1/4 c	60	0	0	0	6	6	15*	2	35	0
RED BEANS											
Eden Foods, organic, canned	1/2 c	100	0.5	0	0	5	<1	0	4	0	+
S&W, canned, Louisiana style	1/2 c	80	0	0	0	5	2	0	4	4	+
RED SNAPPER, broiled	3 oz	109	1	0	0	0	0	0	3	2	+

Food	Portion Size	Calories	Total Fat (g)	Good Fats (g)	Bad Fats (g)	Fiber (g)	Sugars (mg)	Beta-carotene (mcg)	Calcium (%DV)	Vit. C (%DV)	B vit. (0,+,++)
REFRIED BEANS											
Eden Foods											
Black beans, organic	½ c	110	1.5	0	0	7	0	0	4	0	+
Kidney beans, organic	½ c	80	1	0	0	6	0	0	4	0	0
Pinto, organic	½ c	90	1	0	0	7	1	0	4	0	0
Pinto, spicy, organic	½ c	90	1	0	0	7	1	0	4	0	0
Old El Paso											
Fat-free	½ c	100	0	0	0	6	1	0	4	0	0
Fat-free, spicy	½ c	100	0	0	0	6	1	0	4	0	0
Traditional	½ c	100	0.5	0	0	6	1	0	4	0	0
Vegetarian	½ c	100	1	0	0	6	2	0	4	0	0
RHUBARB, raw, diced	1 c	26	0	0	0	2	1	74	10	16	0
RICE											
Long grain, white, prep.	1 c	205	0	0	0	1	0	0	1	0	+
Short grain, white prep.	1 c	242	0	0	0	0	0	0	0	0	+
Carolina, extra long grain white, prep.	¾ c	150	0	0	0	0	0	0	0	0	+
Carolina, gold (parboiled), prep.	1 c	160	0	0	0	<1	0	0	0	0	+
Carolina, jasmine, prep.	¾ c	160	0	0	0	0	0	0	0	0	+
Carolina, long grain brown, prep.	¾ c	150	1	0	0	1	0	0	0	0	+
Uncle Ben's fast & natural brown, prep.	1 c	190	1	0	0	2	0	0	0	3	+
Uncle Ben's long grain & wild, prep.	1 c	200	0	0	0	1	1	0	6	8	+

RICE MIXES

Food	Portion Size	Calories	Total Fat (g)	Good Fats (g)	Bad Fats (g)	Fiber (g)	Sugars (mg)	Beta-carotene (mcg)	Calcium (%DV)	Vit. C (%DV)	B vit. (0,+,++)
Betty Crocker Bowl Appetit											
Cheddar broccoli rice bowl	1	290	7	Na	4.5	2	9	Na	15	0	+
Herb chicken vegetable bowl	1	260	5	Na	2.5	2	2	Na	2	0	+
Teriyaki rice bowl	1	260	3	Na	1.5	2	6	Na	2	0	+
Carolina											
Authentic Spanish, mix	1/5 c	180	0	0	0	1	1	0	0	6	+
Black bean & rice, mix	1/5 c	200	1.5	0	0	5	0	0	6	0	+
Chicken & rice, mix	1/5 c	190	0	0	0	<1	0	0	10	0	+
Classic pilaf, mix	1/5 c	190	0	0	0	1	0	0	0	0	+
Saffron yellow, mix	1/5 c	190	0	0	0	<1	1	0	4	0	+
Spicy yellow, mix	1/5 c	180	0.5	0	0	<1	2	0	2	0	+
Uncle Ben's											
Chicken & herb, prep.	1 c	200	1	0	0	<1	0	0	4	0	Na
Country Inn, Mexican Fiesta, prep.	1 c	200	1	0	0	1	0	0	4	15	+
Country Inn, Oriental fried rice, prep.	1 c	200	1	0	0	1	1	0	2	4	+
Country Inn, rice pilaf, prep.	1 c	200	0.5	0	0	1	1	0	2	0	+
Four cheese, prep.	1 c	190	1	0	0	1	1	0	6	0	+
Parmesan & butter, prep.	1 c	200	1	0	0	<1	0	0	4	0	Na
Roasted chicken, prep.	1 c	200	1	0	0	<1	0	0	4	0	Na
Near East											
Chicken rice pilaf, mix unprep.	1/4 c	190	0.5	0	0	2	1	Na	2	20	Na
Long grain & wild, mix unprep.	1/3 c	190	0.5	0	0	2	0	Na	2	4	Na

Food	Portion Size	Calories	Total Fat (g)	Good Fats (g)	Bad Fats (g)	Fiber (g)	Sugars (mg)	Beta-carotene (mcg)	Calcium (%DV)	Vit. C (%DV)	B vit. (0,+,++)
Rice pilaf toasted almond, mix unprep.	1/4 c	200	3	0	0	2	1	Na	2	0	Na
Sundried tomato & basil, mix unprep.	1/3 c	240	0.5	0	0	2	2	Na	2	8	Na
Rice-A-Roni											
Beef, mix unprep.	1/5 c	230	1	0	0	2	3	Na	2	0	+
Broccoli au gratin, mix unprep.	1/5 c	260	6	Na	3	2	4	Na	6	2	+
Creamy 4 cheese, mix unprep.	1/4 c	210	6	Na	2.5	1	3	Na	4	0	+
Chicken, mix unprep.	1/5 c	230	1	0	0	2	3	Na	2	0	+
Chicken & garlic, mix unprep.	1/5 c	190	0.5	0	0	1	2	Na	2	0	+
Fried, mix unprep.	1/5 c	240	1.5	Na	0	2	4	Na	2	2	+
Herb & butter, mix unprep.	1/5 c	240	1.5	Na	0.5	1	2	Na	2	2	+
Pilaf, mix unprep.	1/5 c	230	1	0	0	2	1	Na	0	0	+
Spanish, mix unprep.	1/5 c	180	0.5	0	0	2	3	Na	2	15	+
RICE BEVERAGES											
Rice Dream, carob	8 oz	150	2.5	1.5	0	<1	26	Na	0	0	0
Rice Dream, chocolate, enriched	8 oz	170	3	2	0	<1	28	Na	30	0	+
Rice Dream, original	8 oz	120	2	1.5	0	0	10	Na	30	0	+
Rice Dream, vanilla	8 oz	130	2	1.5	0	0	12	Na	2	0	0
Rice Dream, vanilla (Heartwise)	8 oz	140	2	1.5	0	3	10	Na	30	0	+
Westbrae, plain	8 oz	100	2.5	1.5	0	0	14	Na	0	0	+
Westbrae, vanilla	8 oz	100	2.5	1.5	0	0	17	Na	25	0	+
RICE CAKES											
Apple cinnamon	1 cake	50	0	0	0	0	3	Na	0	0	0
Butter popped corn	1 cake	35	0	0	0	0	0	0	0	0	0
Caramel corn (Quaker)	1 cake	50	0	0	0	0	3	Na	0	0	0

Food	Portion Size	Calories	Total Fat (g)	Good Fats (g)	Bad Fats (g)	Fiber (g)	Sugars (mg)	Beta-carotene (mcg)	Calcium (%DV)	Vit. C (%DV)	B vit. (0,+,++)
Chocolate crunch	1 cake	60	1	0	0	0	4	Na	0	0	0
Cracker Jack butter toffee (Quaker)	1 cake	60	0.5	0	0	0	4	Na	0	0	0
Maple brown sugar	1 cake	50	1	0	0	1	3	Na	0	0	0
Peanut butter chocolate chip	1 cake	60	1	0	0	0	4	Na	0	0	0
White cheddar	1 cake	45	0.5	0	0	0	1	Na	0	0	0
RICE PUDDING (Also see "Pudding")											
ROCKFISH, Pacific, baked	3 oz	103	2	Na	0	0	0	0	1	0	+
ROLLS (nonsweet)											
Pepperidge Farm											
Carb style, hamburger	1	110	1	0	0	3	1	0	4	0	0
Farmhouse country wheat	1	220	4.5	Na	1	1	6	0	8	0	0
Frankfurter	1	140	2.5	Na	1	1	4	0	6	0	0
Hot & crusty French	1	100	1	Na	0	1	1	0	2	0	0
Hot & crusty 7 grain	1	110	2	Na	0.5	2	3	0	4	0	0
Soft 100% whole wheat Kaiser	1	200	2.5	Na	0.5	3	5	0	6	0	0
Soft country style dinner	1	90	1.5	Na	0	1	3	0	2	0	0
Soft white Kaiser	1	210	2.5	Na	0.5	1	4	0	6	0	0
Pillsbury											
Crescent big & buttery	1	170	10	Na	5	<1	4	0	0	0	0
Crescent big & flaky	1	180	10	Na	5	<1	4	0	0	0	0
Crescent butterflake	1	110	6	Na	3.5	0	2	0	0	0	0
Crescent original	1	110	6	Na	3.5	<1	2	0	0	0	0
Dinner, white quick	1	110	2	Na	1	<1	3	0	0	0	0
Freezer to Microwave, white dinner	1	150	4	Na	2	<1	3	0	0	0	0

Food	Portion Size	Calories	Total Fat (g)	Good Fats (g)	Bad Fats (g)	Fiber (g)	Sugars (mg)	Beta-carotene (mcg)	Calcium (%DV)	Vit. C (%DV)	B vit. (0,+,++)
Freezer to Oven crusty French	1	100	1.5	Na	0	<1	1	0	0	0	0
Freezer to Oven, dinner, garlic	1	140	6	Na	2.5	<1	2	0	0	0	0
Freezer to Oven, dinner, whole wheat	1	90	1	0	0	3	2	0	0	0	0
ROLLS (Sweet)—*Pillsbury*											
Grands! Extra rich cinnamon w/icing	1	320	10	Na	5.5	1	24	0	2	0	0
Grands! Sweet cinnamon w/icing	1	310	9	Na	4.5	1	23	0	2	0	0
Sweet Rolls, caramel	1	170	7	Na	4	<1	10	0	0	0	0
Sweet Rolls, cinnamon w/cream cheese icing	1	150	5	Na	3.5	<1	10	0	0	0	0
Sweet Rolls, cinnamon w/icing, sugar free	1	110	3.5	Na	2	8	0	0	0	0	0
Sweet Rolls, golden homestyle cinnamon	1	130	3	Na	2	<1	9	0	0	0	0
Sweet Rolls, orange w/icing	1	170	7	Na	3.5	<1	10	0	0	0	0
RUTABAGAS, cooked w/o salt, mashed	1 c	93	1	0	0	4	14	2	11	75	+
SALAD DRESSING											
Annie's Naturals											
Artichoke parmesan	2 tbs	130	13	Na	1.5	0	<1	0	2	0	0
Balsamic vinaigrette	2 tbs	100	10	Na	0.5	0	3	0	0	0	0
Thousand island	2 tbs	90	7	Na	1	0	4	0	0	0	0
Woodstock	2 tbs	110	11	Na	1	0	0	0	0	0	0
Kraft											
Catalina fat free	2 tbs	35	0	0	0	1	7	Na	0	0	0
Creamy French	2 tbs	160	15	Na	2.5	0	5	Na	0	0	0
Creamy Italian	2 tbs	110	11	Na	1.5	0	2	Na	0	0	0
Italian fat free	2 tbs	15	0	0	0	0	2	Na	0	0	0

Food	Portion Size	Calories	Total Fat (g)	Good Fats (g)	Bad Fats (g)	Fiber (g)	Sugars (mg)	Beta-carotene (mcg)	Calcium (%DV)	Vit. C (%DV)	B vit. (0,+,++)
Ranch	2 tbs	170	18	Na	3	0	1	Na	0	0	0
Ranch garlic	2 tbs	180	19	Na	3	1	1	Na	0	0	0
Roka blue cheese	2 tbs	130	13	Na	2.5	0	1	Na	0	0	0
Thousand island	2 tbs	120	10	Na	1.5	1	4	Na	0	0	0
Three cheese Italian	2 tbs	130	14	Na	2.5	0	1	Na	0	0	0
Zesty Italian	2 tbs	110	11	Na	1.5	0	2	Na	0	0	0
Kraft—Carb Well											
Classic Caesar	1 tbs	110	11	Na	2	0	0	0	0	0	0
Creamy French	2 tbs	100	11	Na	1.5	0	0	0	0	0	0
Italian	2 tbs	70	10	Na	1	0	0	0	0	0	0
Light buttermilk ranch	2 tbs	60	6	Na	1	0	0	0	0	0	0
Ranch	2 tbs	110	11	Na	1.5	0	0	0	0	0	0
Roka blue cheese	2 tbs	120	13	Na	2	0	0	0	0	0	0
Kraft—Light Done Right											
Creamy French	2 tbs	80	4.5	0	0.5	0	6	0	0	0	0
Italian	2 tbs	40	3	0	0.5	0	1	0	0	0	0
Ranch	2 tbs	80	7	0	0.5	0	1	0	0	0	0
Zesty Italian, reduced fat	2 tbs	25	1.5	0	0	0	2	0	0	0	0
Kraft—Special Collection											
Caesar Italian w/oregano	2 tbs	100	10	Na	1.5	0	1	0	2	0	0
Creamy poppy seed	2 tbs	130	10	Na	2	0	8	0	0	0	0
Greek vinaigrette	2 tbs	11	Na	1.5	0	1	0	0	0	0	0
Italian pesto	2 tbs	70	5	Na	0.5	0	2	0	0	0	0

Food	Portion Size	Calories	Total Fat (g)	Good Fats (g)	Bad Fats (g)	Fiber (g)	Sugars (mg)	Beta-carotene (mcg)	Calcium (%DV)	Vit. C (%DV)	B vit. (0,+,++)
Sundried tomato	2 tbs	60	5	Na	0.5	0	3	0	0	0	0
Tangy tomato bacon	2 tbs	130	10	Na	1.5	0	7	0	0	0	0
Newman's Own											
Caesar	2 tbs	150	16	Na	1.5	0	1	0	2	0	0
Olive oil & vinegar	2 tbs	150	16	Na	2.5	0	0	0	0	0	0
Ranch	2 tbs	140	15	Na	2	0	2	0	0	0	0
2000 island	2 tbs	140	14	Na	2	0	3	0	0	0	0
Three cheese balsamic	2 tbs	100	11	Na	1.5	0	1	0	2	2	0
Seven Seas											
Creamy Italian	2 tbs	110	12	Na	2	0	2	0	0	0	0
Green goddess	2 tbs	130	13	Na	2	0	1	0	0	0	0
Red wine vinaigrette	2 tbs	90	9	Na	0.5	0	2	0	0	0	0
Viva Italian	2 tbs	90	9	Na	1.5	0	1	0	0	0	0
Viva Italian, reduced fat	2 tbs	45	4	Na	0.5	0	1	0	0	0	0
South Beach Diet											
Italian w/extra olive oil	2 tbs	60	4.5	Na	0	0	2	0	0	0	0
Ranch	2 tbs	70	7	Na	1	0	0	0	0	0	0
Wishbone											
Chunky blue cheese	2 tbs	150	15	Na	2.5	0	1	0	0	0	0
Creamy Caesar	2 tbs	170	18	Na	3	0	<1	0	0	0	0
Deluxe French	2 tbs	120	11	Na	1.5	0	5	0	0	0	0
Garlic ranch	2 tbs	140	15	Na	2	0	<1	0	0	0	0
Russian	2 tbs	120	6	Na	1	0	60	0	0	4	0

Food	Portion Size	Calories	Total Fat (g)	Good Fats (g)	Bad Fats (g)	Fiber (g)	Sugars (mg)	Beta-carotene (mcg)	Calcium (%DV)	Vit. C (%DV)	B vit. (0,+,++)
Sweet 'n spicy	2 tbs	130	12	Na	2	0	5	0	0	2	0
Thousand Island	2 tbs	130	12	Na	2	0	4	0	0	0	0
Wishbone—Fat Free											
Chunky blue cheese	2 tbs	35	0	0	0	<1	3	0	0	0	0
Italian	2 tbs	20	0	0	0	0	3	0	0	4	0
Ranch	2 tbs	30	0	0	0	<1	3	0	0	0	0
Wishbone—Just2Good											
Blue cheese	2 tbs	50	2	Na	0.5	0	2	0	0	0	0
Creamy Caesar	2 tbs	50	2	Na	0.5	0	2	0	0	0	0
Deluxe French	2 tbs	50	2	Na	0	<1	6	0	0	0	0
Honey Dijon	2 tbs	50	2	Na	0	<1	6	0	0	0	0
Ranch	2 tbs	40	2	Na	0	0	2	0	0	0	0
Thousand Island	2 tbs	50	2	Na	0	0	5	0	0	0	0
Wishbone—Salad Spritzers											
Balsamic Breeze, Italian vinaigrette, and Red wine mist	10 sprays	10	1	0	0	0	1	0	0	0	0
Wishbone—Western											
Bacon flavor	2 tbs	140	11	Na	1.5	0	10	0	0	0	0
Blue cheese	2 tbs	140	12	Na	2	0	9	0	0	0	0
Fat-free	2 tbs	50	0	0	0	0	11	0	0	0	0
Original	2 tbs	160	12	Na	1.5	0	11	0	0	0	0
SALAMI											
Louis Rich turkey salami	1 oz	41	3	1	1	0	0	Na	1	0	0
Oscar Mayer, cotto	1 oz	70	6	3	2	0	0	0	1	0	0

Food	Portion Size	Calories	Total Fat (g)	Good Fats (g)	Bad Fats (g)	Fiber (g)	Sugars (mg)	Beta-carotene (mcg)	Calcium (%DV)	Vit. C (%DV)	B vit. (0,+,++)
Oscar Mayer, cotto beef	1 oz	60	4.5	2	2	0	0	0	0	0	0
Oscar Mayer, genoa	1 oz	105	9	4.5	3	0	0	Na	1	0	0
Oscar Mayer, hard	1 oz	100	8	4	3	0	0	5.4	0	0	0
SALMON											
Canned, blueback (Bumblebee)	2.2 oz	110	7	Na	1.5	0	0	0	10	0	+
Canned, keta (Bumblebee)	2.2 oz	90	4	Na	1	0	0	0	10	0	+
Canned, pink (Bumblebee)	2.2 oz	90	5	1	1	0	0	0	10	0	+
Canned, red (Bumblebee)	2.2 oz	110	7	1	1.5	0	0	0	10	0	+
Canned, pink (Chicken of the Sea), skinless	2 oz	60	2	1	1	0	0	0	0	0	+
Canned, trad. red (Chicken of the Sea)	2 oz	110	7	1	2	0	0	0	10	0	+
Fresh, Atlantic wild, cooked dry	3 oz	155	7	3.5	1	0	0	0	1	5	+
Fresh, Chinook wild, cooked dry	3 oz	196	11	5	3	0	0	0	2	5	+
Smoked Pacific (Chicken of the Sea)	1 pkg	120	3.5	Na	1	0	1	0	2	2	+
Steak w/orange glaze (Chicken of the Sea)	1 pkg	170	1.5	0	0.5	0	12	0	2	0	+
SALSA											
Muir Glen organic, black bean & corn	2 tbs	20	0	0	0	<1	<1	0	0	6	0
Muir Glen organic, mild	2 tbs	10	0	0	0	0	1	0	0	8	0
Newman's Own black bean & corn	2 tbs	20	0	0	0	2	1	0	2	0	0
Newman's Own, mango	2 tbs	20	0	0	0	2	1	0	2	0	0
Newman's Own, natural bandito mild	2 tbs	10	0	0	0	1	1	0	2	0	0
Newman's Own, peach	2 tbs	25	0	0	0	<1	5	0	0	0	0
Newman's Own, tequila lime	2 tbs	15	0	0	0	0	2	0	2	0	0
Old El Paso, cheese 'n salsa medium	2 tbs	40	3	Na	1	0	0	0	2	0	0
Old El Paso, thick 'n chunky, mild	2 tbs	10	0	0	0	0	1	0	0	0	0

Food	Portion Size	Calories	Total Fat (g)	Good Fats (g)	Bad Fats (g)	Fiber (g)	Sugars (mg)	Beta-carotene (mcg)	Calcium (%DV)	Vit. C (%DV)	B vit. (0,+,++)
Pace, chunky	2 tbs	10	0	0	0	<1	2	0	0	0	0
Pace, lime & garlic chunky	2 tbs	15	0	0	0	<1	2	0	0	3	0
SARDINES											
Bumblebee, in mustard	3.75 oz	130	6	Na	1.5	1	1	0	15	0	+
Bumblebee, in soya oil	3.75 oz	130	9	Na	2	0	0	0	10	0	+
Bumblebee, in water	3.75 oz	120	7	Na	2	0	0	0	10	0	+
Chicken of the Sea, smoked in oil	1 can	190	14	3.5	6	0	0	0	20	0	+
Chicken of the Sea, in tomato	1 can	130	6	Na	2	2	2	18*	30	4	+
Crown Prince, brisling in mustard	1 can	210	16	Na	6	<1	0	Na	20	2	+
Crown Prince, brisling in soy oil	1 can	200	16	Na	4.5	<1	0	Na	20	0	+
Crown Prince, brisling in tomato	1 can	210	16	Na	6	<1	2	Na	20	0	+
SAUCES											
A-1 Sauce											
Jamaican jerk steak sauce	2 tbs	25	0.5	0	0	0	4	0	0	0	0
New York steak sauce	2 tbs	20	0	0	0	0	4	0	0	0	0
Teriyaki steak sauce	2 tbs	20	0	0	0	0	4	0	0	0	0
Kraft											
Cocktail	2 tbs	60	0.5	0	0	1	9	Na	0	4	0
Coleslaw maker	2 tbs	110	9	Na	1.5	0	6	0	0	0	0
Sweet & sour	2 tbs	60	0	0	0	0	12	0	0	2	0
Tarter sauce	2 tbs	70	6	Na	1	0	3	0	0	0	0
Old El Paso											
Enchilada, mild	¼ c	25	1	0	0	0	1	0	0	0	0

Food	Portion Size	Calories	Total Fat (g)	Good Fats (g)	Bad Fats (g)	Fiber (g)	Sugars (mg)	Beta-carotene (mcg)	Calcium (%DV)	Vit. C (%DV)	B vit. (0,+,++)
Taco sauce, mild	1 tbs	5	0	0	0	0	1	0	0	0	0
Zesty ranch sauce	2 tbs	70	6	Na	1	0	1	0	0	0	0
SAUERKRAUT											
Del Monte	2 tbs	0	0	0	0	<1	0	0	0	2	0
Del Monte, Bavarian	2 tbs	15	0	0	0	0	3	0	0	2	0
Eden Foods, organic	½ c	25	0	0	0	3	1	9*	4	20	0
S&W	2 tbs	0	0	0	0	<1	0	0	0	2	0
SAUSAGE											
Armour Brown & Serve, lite original	3 links	120	8	Na	3	0	1	Na	4	0	Na
Armour Brown & Serve, turkey	3 links	120	8	Na	2.5	0	1	Na	4	0	Na
Italian pork	3 oz	230	18	8	6	0	1	0	1	0	+
Italian sweet	3 oz	125	7	3	3	0	0	0	2	0	0
Lightlife, Gimme lean sausage style (soy)	2 oz	50	0	0	0	2	1	0	0	0	0
Lightlife, Smart country breakfast links	2 links	100	3.5	Na	0.5	4	2	0	0	0	0
Oscar Mayer, pork sausage links	2 links	130	11	6	4	0	0	0	0	0	0
Oscar Mayer, turkey sausage, original	3 oz	120	8	Na	2.5	0	0	0	1	0	Na
Polish sausage, beef & chicken	2 oz	259	19	10	8	0	0	0	0	0	+
SESAME											
Arrowhead Mills, tahini (sesame spread)	2 tbs	190	18	6	2.5	<1	1	0	4	0	0
Maranatha tahini butter, no salt, roasted	2 tbs	210	16	6	2	3	0	0	2	0	+
SHAD, American, cooked dry	3 oz	214	15	Na	0	0	0	0	5	0	
SHERBET											
Dreyer's, berry rainbow or tropical rainbow	½ c	130	1.5	Na	0.5	0	23	0	4	0	0
Dreyer's, key lime	½ c	130	1.5	Na	0.5	0	23	0	4	0	0

Food	Portion Size	Calories	Total Fat (g)	Good Fats (g)	Bad Fats (g)	Fiber (g)	Sugars (mg)	Beta-carotene (mcg)	Calcium (%DV)	Vit. C (%DV)	B vit. (0,+,++)
Dreyer's, orange cream	½ c	130	2	Na	1	0	19	0	4	0	0
Dreyer's, raspberry or strawberry	½ c	130	1	Na	0.5	0	22	0	4	0	0
Dreyer's, swiss orange	½ c	150	3	Na	2.5	0	25	0	4	0	0
SHRIMP											
Canned, regular (Bumblebee)	¼ c	40	0	0	0	0	1	0	6	0	0
Frozen, premium, cooked (Chicken of the Sea), large, tail on	3 oz	80	1	0	0	0	0	0	2	0	0
Frozen, premium, raw (Chicken of the Sea)	4 oz	120	2	Na	0	0	0	0	6	0	0
SNACK MIX											
Chex, bold party blend	½ c	140	6	Na	1.5	<1	2	0	0	0	0
Chex mix, cheddar	⅔ c	130	4	Na	1	<1	3	0	2	0	0
Chex mix, honey nut	½ c	130	4	Na	0.5	<1	5	0	2	0	0
Chex mix, hot 'n spicy	⅔ c	130	4	Na	1.5	1	2	0	0	0	0
Chex mix, peanut lovers	½ c	140	6	Na	1	1	2	0	0	0	0
Chex mix, summer ranch	⅔ c	120	3	Na	0.5	<1	3	0	0	0	0
Chex mix, traditional	⅔ c	130	4	Na	0.5	1	2	0	0	0	0
Chex trail mix	½ c	140	4.5	Na	1.5	1	7	0	0	0	0
Chex chocolate peanut butter	⅔ c	150	5	Na	1.5	<1	9	0	0	0	0
Chocolate turtle	⅔ c	150	5	Na	2	<1	10	0	0	0	0
Gardetto's Italian cheese blend	½ c	140	5	Na	2	<1	2	0	0	0	0
Gardetto's mustard pretzel mix	½ c	130	2	Na	0	1	<1	0	0	0	0
Gardetto's snack mix, original	½ c	150	6	Na	3	1	1	0	0	0	0

Food	Portion Size	Calories	Total Fat (g)	Good Fats (g)	Bad Fats (g)	Fiber (g)	Sugars (mg)	Beta-carotene (mcg)	Calcium (%DV)	Vit. C (%DV)	B vit. (0,+,++)
Nabisco, cheddar	1 oz	130	4.5	Na	1	1	0	0	0	0	0
Nabisco, traditional	1 oz	130	5	Na	1	1	2	0	2	0	0
Planter's trail mix, fruit & nut	1 oz	140	9	Na	2.5	2	9	Na	0	0	Na
Planter's trail mix, golden nut crunch	1 oz	160	11	Na	2	2	7	Na	4	0	Na
Planter's trail mix, mixed nuts & raisins	1 oz	150	11	Na	1.5	2	6	Na	2	0	Na
Planter's trail mix, nut & chocolate	1 oz	160	10	Na	2.5	2	13	Na	2	0	Na
Planter's trail mix, spicy nuts	1 oz	150	10	Na	1.5	2	1	Na	2	0	Na
SOFT DRINKS											
Hansen's Natural sodas											
Ginger ale	12 oz	140	0	0	0	0	37	0	0	0	0
Grapefruit	12 oz	160	0	0	0	0	43	0	0	0	0
Key lime	12 oz	130	0	0	0	0	36	0	0	0	0
Kiwi strawberry	12 oz	130	0	0	0	0	36	0	0	0	0
Mandarin lime	12 oz	130	0	0	0	0	35	0	0	0	0
Orange mango	12 oz	160	0	0	0	0	43	0	0	0	0
Root beer	12 oz	160	0	0	0	0	43	0	0	0	0
Vanilla cola	12 oz	160	0	0	0	0	43	0	0	0	0
IBC											
Black cherry	12 oz	180	0	0	0	0	48	0	0	0	0
Cream	12 oz	180	0	0	0	0	48	0	0	0	0
Root beer	12 oz	160	0	0	0	0	43	0	0	0	0
Mountain Dew											
Amp	8 oz	110	0	0	0	0	29	0	0	0	0
Baja blast	8 oz	110	0	0	0	0	29	0	0	0	0

Food	Portion Size	Calories	Total Fat (g)	Good Fats (g)	Bad Fats (g)	Fiber (g)	Sugars (mg)	Beta-carotene (mcg)	Calcium (%DV)	Vit. C (%DV)	B vit. (0,+,++)
Livewire	8 oz	110	0	0	0	0	31	0	0	0	0
MDX	8 oz	120	0	0	0	0	32	0	0	0	0
Regular and caffeine free	8 oz	110	0	0	0	0	31	0	0	0	0
Pepsi brands											
Diet, all	8 oz	0	0	0	0	0	0	0	0	0	0
Regular and caffeine free	8 oz	100	0	0	0	0	27	0	0	0	0
Sierra Mist	8 oz	100	0	0	0	0	26	0	0	0	0
Twist	8 oz	100	0	0	0	0	27	0	0	0	0
Wild cherry	8 oz	110	0	0	0	0	29	0	0	0	0
Vanilla	8 oz	110	0	0	0	0	28	0	0	0	0
Schweppes											
Club soda	8 oz	0	0	0	0	0	0	0	0	0	0
Ginger ale	8 oz	80	0	0	0	0	22	0	0	0	0
Tonic water	8 oz	90	0	0	0	0	22	0	0	0	0
SORBET											
Ben & Jerry's											
Berried Treasure	½ c	110	0	0	0	1	24	0	0	6	0
Jamaican Me Crazy	½ c	130	0	0	0	<1	28	0	0	6	0
Strawberry kiwi	½ c	110	0	0	0	1	24	0	0	8	0
Häagen-Dazs											
Chocolate	½ c	130	0.5	0	0	2	20	0	0	0	0
Mango	½ c	120	0	0	0	0	36	0	0	0	0
Strawberry	½ c	120	0	0	0	<1	30	0	0	15	0

Food	Portion Size	Calories	Total Fat (g)	Good Fats (g)	Bad Fats (g)	Fiber (g)	Sugars (mg)	Beta-carotene (mcg)	Calcium (%DV)	Vit. C (%DV)	B vit. (0,+,++)
Tropical	½ c	150	0	0	0	0	38	0	0	4	0
Zesty lemon	½ c	110	0	0	0	<1	29	0	2	4	0
SOUPS											
Campbell's											
Bean w/bacon	½ c	170	4	Na	1.5	8	4	0	6	0	Na
Beef noodle	½ c	70	2.5	Na	0.5	<1	1	0	0	0	Na
Beef w/vegetables & barley	½ c	90	1.5	0	1	3	2	0	0	0	Na
Black bean	½ c	110	1.5	Na	0.5	6	5	Na	4	0	Na
Broccoli cheese	½ c	100	4.5	Na	2	0	2	Na	4	2	Na
Chicken & dumplings	½ c	70	2.5	Na	1	1	1	Na	0	0	Na
Chicken & stars	½ c	70	2	Na	0.5	1	1	Na	0	0	Na
Chicken gumbo	½ c	60	1	0	0.5	1	2	Na	2	0	Na
Chicken noodle	½ c	60	2	1	0.5	0	0	0	1	0	+
Chicken vegetable	½ c	80	1	0	0.5	2	3	Na	2	0	Na
Chicken won ton	½ c	60	1	0	0.5	0	1	Na	0	0	Na
Cream of broccoli, 98% fat free	½ c	70	2	Na	0.5	2	1	Na	2	0	Na
Cream of celery	½ c	90	6	Na	1	3	1	Na	2	0	Na
Cream of chicken	½ c	120	8	Na	2.5	2	1	Na	0	0	Na
Cream of chicken, 98% fat free	½ c	70	2.5	Na	1	1	1	Na	0	0	Na
Cream of mushroom	½ c	100	6	Na	1.5	2	1	Na	0	0	Na
Cream of potato	½ c	90	2	Na	1	2	1	Na	0	0	Na
Cream of shrimp	½ c	90	5	Na	1	1	0	Na	0	0	Na
Creamy tomato ranchero	½ c	130	6	Na	2	4	4	Na	2	2	Na
Fiesta chili beef	½ c	170	5	Na	2	8	5	Na	4	0	Na

Food	Portion Size	Calories	Total Fat (g)	Good Fats (g)	Bad Fats (g)	Fiber (g)	Sugars (mg)	Beta-carotene (mcg)	Calcium (%DV)	Vit. C (%DV)	B vit. (0,+,++)
Fiesta nacho cheese	½ c	120	8	Na	4	1	2	Na	8	0	Na
French onion	½ c	45	1.5	0	1	1	4	Na	2	0	Na
Golden mushroom	½ c	80	3.5	0	1	1	1	Na	0	0	Na
Goldfish meatball	½ c	180	2.5	Na	1.5	2	1	Na	0	0	Na
Green pea	½ c	180	3	Na	1	11	6	Na	2	0	Na
Hearty vegetable w/pasta	½ c	90	0.5	0	0	2	8	Na	2	2	Na
Manhattan clam chowder	½ c	70	0.5	0	0.5	2	2	Na	2	2	Na
Minestrone	½ c	90	1	0	0.5	3	3	Na	2	0	Na
New England clam chowder	½ c	90	2.5	Na	0.5	1	1	Na	2	0	Na
New England clam chowder, 98% fat free	½ c	80	2	Na	0.5	2	1	0	0	0	Na
Old fashioned vegetable	½ c	80	1.5	0	0.5	2	3	Na	2	0	Na
Pepper pot	½ c	90	4	Na	1.5	1	1	Na	2	0	Na
Scotch broth	½ c	90	4	Na	1.5	1	1	Na	2	0	Na
Split pea w/ham & bacon	½ c	180	3.5	Na	2	5	4	Na	2	0	Na
Tomato noodle	½ c	120	0.5	0	0	2	3	Na	0	0	Na
Tomato	½ c	90	0	0	0	1	12	Na	0	10	Na
Vegetable beef	½ c	90	1	0	0.5	3	2	Na	0	10	Na
Vegetarian vegetable	½ c	90	0.5	0	0	2	6	Na	2	0	Na
Campbell's Chunky											
Baked potato w/cheddar & bacon	1 c	160	6	Na	1	2	3	Na	4	0	Na
Baked potato w/steak & cheese	1 c	210	10	Na	2.5	3	3	Na	2	0	Na
Beef w/country vegetable	1 c	150	2.5	Na	1	4	4	Na	2	0	Na
Chicken & dumplings	1 c	180	7	Na	2	4	3	Na	2	0	Na

Food	Portion Size	Calories	Total Fat (g)	Good Fats (g)	Bad Fats (g)	Fiber (g)	Sugars (mg)	Beta-carotene (mcg)	Calcium (%DV)	Vit. C (%DV)	B vit. (0,+,++)
Chicken mushroom chowder	1 c	210	12	Na	3	3	3	Na	2	0	Na
Grilled chicken & sausage gumbo	1 c	140	2.5	Na	1	3	4	Na	2	0	Na
Hearty bean & ham	1 c	180	2	Na	0.5	8	5	Na	6	2	Na
Hearty beef barley	1 c	170	2.5	Na	1	4	5	Na	2	2	Na
Honey roasted ham w/potatoes	1 c	130	2.5	Na	1	3	7	Na	4	2	Na
New England clam chowder	1 c	210	9	Na	1	5	2	Na	2	0	Na
Pepper steak	1 c	120	1.5	0	0.5	3	4	Na	2	2	Na
Savory pot roast	1 c	120	1.5	0	1	3	4	Na	2	2	Na
Savory vegetable	1 c	110	1	0	0.5	4	6	Na	4	2	Na
Split pea & ham	1 c	170	2.5	Na	1	4	5	Na	2	4	Na
Steak & potato	1 c	130	2	Na	0.5	2	2	Na	0	0	Na
Turkey pot pie	1 c	180	7	Na	2	4	3	Na	2	0	Na
Campbell's Chunky Microwaveable											
Beef w/country vegetables	1 c	150	3	Na	1.5	5	3	Na	2	2	Na
Chicken & dumplings	1 c	190	9	Na	2	3	2	Na	2	0	Na
New England clam chowder	1 c	200	12	Na	2.5	3	2	Na	8	0	Na
Sirloin burger w/country vegetables	1 c	160	4	Na	2	4	4	Na	2	0	Na
Campbell's Healthy Request											
Chicken noodle	½ c	60	2	Na	0.5	1	1	Na	0	0	Na
Cream of celery	½ c	70	2	Na	0	1	2	Na	0	0	Na
Cream of mushroom	½ c	70	2	Na	0.5	1	2	Na	10	0	Na
Minestrone	½ c	80	0.5	0	0	3	4	Na	4	0	Na
Vegetable beef	½ c	100	1	0	0	3	5	Na	2	0	Na

Food	Portion Size	Calories	Total Fat (g)	Good Fats (g)	Bad Fats (g)	Fiber (g)	Sugars (mg)	Beta-carotene (mcg)	Calcium (%DV)	Vit. C (%DV)	B vit. (0,+,++)
Campbell's Select											
Beef w/roasted barley	1 c	130	1	0	0.5	2	4	Na	2	0	Na
Chicken vegetable medley	1 c	110	0.5	0	0.5	2	4	Na	2	0	Na
Creamy chicken alfredo	1 c	180	7	Na	1	2	1	Na	4	0	Na
Italian style wedding	1 c	120	3	Na	1.5	2	3	Na	4	0	Na
Minestrone	1 c	100	0.5	0	0	3	5	Na	4	0	Na
New England clam chowder, 98% fat free	1 c	110	1.5	Na	0	2	2	Na	4	4	Na
Potato broccoli cheese	1 c	120	4	Na	1	4	2	Na	2	2	Na
Roasted chicken w/rotini	1 c	100	0.5	0	0.5	2	2	Na	6	0	Na
Savory lentil	1 c	140	0.5	0	0.5	6	5	Na	4	0	Na
Split pea w/roasted ham	1 c	160	1	0	0	5	5	Na	4	0	Na
Tomato garden	1 c	100	0.5	0	0.5	2	12	Na	4	0	Na
Vegetable medley	1 c	100	0.5	0	0	3	6	Na	4	0	Na
Campbell's Soup at Hand											
Blended vegetable medley	1 cont	100	1.5	Na	0.5	4	9	Na	2	50	Na
Chicken & stars	1 cont	60	1.5	0	0.5	2	1	Na	0	0	Na
Cream of broccoli	1 cont	150	7	Na	2	7	3	Na	2	0	Na
Velvety potato	1 cont	160	7	Na	1	4	5	Na	2	0	Na
Imagine											
Crab bisque	8 oz	130	5	Na	3	0	4	Na	15	10	Na
Lobster bisque	8 oz	130	5	Na	3	0	4	Na	15	10	Na
Creamy broccoli, organic	8 oz	60	1.5	Na	0	2	3	Na	2	0	Na
Creamy butternut squash, organic	1 c	90	2	Na	0	2	7	Na	4	4	Na
Creamy chicken, organic	1 c	70	1.5	Na	0	1	1	Na	2	8	Na

Food	Portion Size	Calories	Total Fat (g)	Good Fats (g)	Bad Fats (g)	Fiber (g)	Sugars (mg)	Beta-carotene (mcg)	Calcium (%DV)	Vit. C (%DV)	B vit. (0,+,++)
Creamy sweet corn, organic	1 c	120	3	Na	0.6	3	9	Na	2	0	Na
Creamy sweet potato, organic	1 c	110	1.5	Na	0	1	2	Na	2	35	Na
Creamy tomato basil, organic	1 c	90	1.5	Na	0	2	7	Na	4	0	Na
Progresso—50% less sodium											
Chicken gumbo	1 c	110	1.5	0.5	0.5	2	2	80*	2	6	0
Chicken noodle	1 c	90	1.5	0	0	1	2	Na	2	2	0
Garden vegetable	1 c	100	0	0	0	3	4	Na	4	6	0
Progresso—Rich & Hearty											
Beef barley vegetable	1 c	130	1	0	0.5	3	4	400*	2	0	0
Chicken corn chowder	1 c	210	9	2	2.5	2	5	1600*	2	8	0
Chicken & homestyle noodles	1 c	110	2	0.5	0.5	1	1	1200*	2	0	0
Chicken pot pie style	1 c	170	6	Na	1.5	2	3	Na	2	0	0
New England clam chowder	1 c	190	9	Na	2	2	2	Na	2	6	+
Steak & homestyle noodles	1 c	120	3	Na	1	1	3	Na	0	0	0
Steak & sautéed mushrooms	1 c	110	2	Na	0.5	1	3	Na	0	0	0
Progresso—Traditional											
Beef & baked potato	1 c	100	2.5	0.5	1	1	2	Na	2	0	Na
Beef & mushroom	1 c	100	1	0	0	2	4	Na	2	6	Na
Chicken cheese enchilada, Carb Monitor	1 c	170	12	0.5	4	<1	2	Na	6	6	0
Chicken noodle, 99% fat free	1 c	100	2	0.5	0.5	1	1	Na	2	0	0
Chicken vegetable, Carb Monitor	1 c	70	2	Na	1	1	2	900*	2	0	0
New England clam chowder	1 c	190	10	Na	2.5	2	2	Na	2	6	+
New England clam chowder, 99% fat free	1 c	120	2	Na	0	2	2	Na	0	0	+

Food	Portion Size	Calories	Total Fat (g)	Good Fats (g)	Bad Fats (g)	Fiber (g)	Sugars (mg)	Beta-carotene (mcg)	Calcium (%DV)	Vit. C (%DV)	B vit. (0,+,++)
Split pea w/ham	1 c	150	1	0	0.5	4	4	Na	2	0	Na
Turkey noodle	1 c	80	1.5	0	0	1	1	Na	0	0	Na
Tuscan meatball, Carb Monitor	1 c	100	5	Na	2.5	1	2	Na	6	0	0
Progresso—Vegetable Classics											
Creamy mushroom	1 c	130	10	Na	3	2	2	Na	0	0	0
French onion	1 c	50	1.5	Na	0.5	<1	3	Na	0	2	Na
Garden vegetable	1 c	90	0	Na	0	3	3	Na	0	0	Na
Lentil	1 c	150	2	Na	0	5	1	Na	4	0	Na
Minestrone	1 c	110	2	1	0.5	1	0	0	3	1	Na
Tomato basil	1 c	160	3	0.5	0.5	1	16	Na	2	10	Na
Vegetable	1 c	80	0.5	0	0	2	3	Na	2	0	Na
Vegetable Italiano	1 c	100	2	0	0.5	3	7	Na	2	0	Na
Vegetarian vegetable w/barley	1 c	100	0.5	0	0	4	4	Na	2	0	Na
Westbrae Natural											
Alabama black bean gumbo	1 c	140	0	0	0	6	6	Na	6	2	Na
Hearty Milano minestrone	1 c	120	0	0	0	6	4	Na	8	4	Na
Mediterranean lentil	1 c	140	0	0	0	10	5	Na	4	2	Na
Old world split pea	1 c	150	0	0	0	6	5	Na	2	2	Na
Santa Fe vegetable	1 c	160	0	0	0	8	5	Na	6	10	Na
Tuscany tomato	¾ c	70	0	0	0	0	12	Na	2	25	Na
SOUR CREAM											
Breakstone											
Fat-free	2 tbs	30	0	0	0	0	2	0	4	0	0
Reduced fat	2 tbs	40	3	0	2	0	2	0	4	0	0

Food	Portion Size	Calories	Total Fat (g)	Good Fats (g)	Bad Fats (g)	Fiber (g)	Sugars (mg)	Beta-carotene (mcg)	Calcium (%DV)	Vit. C (%DV)	B vit. (0,+,++)
Daisy											
Light	2 tbs	40	2.5	0	2	0	2	0	4	0	0
No fat	2 tbs	20	0	0	0	0	1	0	4	0	0
Regular	2 tbs	60	5	Na	3.5	0	1	0	2	0	0
Knudsen											
Fat free	2 tbs	30	0	0	0	0	2	0	6	0	0
Hampshire	2 tbs	60	6	Na	3.5	0	1	0	2	0	0
Light	2 tbs	30	2	Na	1	0	2	0	4	0	0
SOY BEVERAGES											
Edensoy											
Carob, organic	8 oz	170	4	2.5	0.5	<1	14	Na	8	0	+
Chocolate, organic	8 oz	180	4	2.5	1	<1	15	900*	10	0	+
Original	8 oz	140	5	2	0.5	<1	7	0	10	0	+
Extra original	8 oz	130	4	2.5	0.5	<1	7	0	20	0	+
Light original	8 oz	100	2	1	0	0	10	0	10	0	+
Vanilla	8 oz	150	3	1.5	0.5	<1	16	0	8	0	0
Vanilla, extra	8 oz	150	3	2	0	<1	15	0	20	0	+
Vanilla, light	8 oz	110	1	0.5	0	0	12	0	10	0	0
Pacific											
Plain, low fat, organic	8 oz	70	2.5	Na	0	1	6	0	2	0	Na
Ultra plain, organic	8 oz	120	4	Na	0.5	1	8	0	50	0	+
Ultra vanilla, organic	8 oz	130	4	Na	0.5	1	10	0	50	0	+
Unsweetened original	8 oz	90	4.5	1.5	0.5	2	2	0	2	0	Na
Vanilla, low fat	8 oz	80	2.5	Na	0	<1	6	0	2	0	Na

Food	Portion Size	Calories	Total Fat (g)	Good Fats (g)	Bad Fats (g)	Fiber (g)	Sugars (mg)	Beta-carotene (mcg)	Calcium (%DV)	Vit. C (%DV)	B vit. (0,+,++)
Silk											
Chai	8 oz	130	3.35	Na	0.5	0	14	Na	30	0	+
Chocolate	8 oz	140	3.5	1	0.5	2	19	900*	30	0	+
Chocolate, light	8 oz	120	1.5	1	0	2	19	900*	30	0	+
Enhanced	8 oz	110	5	1	0.5	1	6	Na	35	35	‡‡
Plain	8 oz	100	4	1	0.5	1	6	0	30	0	+
Smoothie, blueberry or mango (Silk Live!)	1 cont	230	4	1	0.5	3	35	0	35	25	‡‡
Smoothie, peach (Silk Live!)	1 cont	220	4	1	0.5	3	32	0	35	25	‡‡
Vanilla, light	8 oz	80	2	0.5	0	1	7	0	30	0	+
Very vanilla	8 oz	130	4	1	0.5	1	16	Na	35	35	+
SOYBEANS (Also see "Tofu")											
Cascadian Farm, edamame	2/3 c	120	5	Na	0.5	3	2	Na	10	20	+
Fresh, cooked, mature, no salt	1 c	298	15	Na	2	10	5	9	17	4	+
Roasted, no salt (NOW)	1/3 c	150	6	Na	1.5	4	1	Na	6	0	+
SPAGHETTI (Also see "Pasta")											
SPAGHETTI SQUASH, cooked, no salt	1 c	42	0	0	0	2	4	91	3	9	0
SPINACH											
Fresh, cooked, drained	1 c	41	0	0	0	4	1	11318	24	29	+
Fresh, raw	1 c	7	0	0	0	1	0	1688	2	14	0
Bird's Eye, chopped or leaf, frozen	1/3 c	30	0	0	0	1	0	7000*	8	2	0
Bird's Eye, creamed w/real cream	1/2 c	100	7	Na	3	1	0	Na	10	2	0
Green Giant, frozen, no sauce	1/2 c	25	0	0	0	1	0	6800*	6	2	0
Green Giant, frozen, creamed	1/2 c	70	2.5	Na	1.5	1	4	Na	10	0	0

Food	Portion Size	Calories	Total Fat (g)	Good Fats (g)	Bad Fats (g)	Fiber (g)	Sugars (mg)	Beta-carotene (mcg)	Calcium (%DV)	Vit. C (%DV)	B vit. (0,+,++)
Green Giant, frozen, cut leaf w/butter	½ c	30	1	0	0	2	1	6800*	8	8	0
S&W, canned, leaf	½ c	30	0	0	0	2	0	5881*	10	25	0
SQUASH (see specific types)											
STRAWBERRIES, fresh, raw, sliced	1 c	49	0	0	0	3	8	11	2	162	0
Cascadian Farm, frozen	1 c	45	0	0	0	3	7	40	2	102	0
STUFFING											
Pepperidge Farm											
Corn bread	¾ c	170	2	Na	0	2	2	0	4	0	0
Cube	¾ c	140	1	Na	0	2	2	0	4	0	0
One step chicken	½ c	160	4	Na	1	2	2	0	2	0	0
One step turkey	½ c	170	7	Na	1	1	2	0	2	0	0
Sage & onion	¾ c	140	1	0	0	3	3	Na	6	0	0
Stove Top											
Chicken	⅙ box	110	1	0	0	1	3	0	0	0	0
Chicken, lower sodium	⅙ box	110	1	0	0	1	3	0	0	0	0
Chicken w/whole wheat	⅕ box	100	1.5	Na	0	3	2	0	0	0	0
Cornbread one step	⅛ box	120	3	Na	0	1	3	0	0	0	0
Homestyle herb one step	⅛ box	110	2.5	Na	0	1	3	0	0	0	0
Turkey	⅙ box	110	1	0	0	1	3	0	0	0	0
SUGAR											
Brown	1 tsp	11	0	0	0	0	3	0	0	0	0
Powdered	1 tsp	10	0	0	0	0	3	0	0	0	0
White, granulated	1 tsp	15	0	0	0	0	4	0	0	0	0

Food	Portion Size	Calories	Total Fat (g)	Good Fats (g)	Bad Fats (g)	Fiber (g)	Sugars (mg)	Beta-carotene (mcg)	Calcium (%DV)	Vit. C (%DV)	B vit. (0,+,++)
SUNFLOWER SEEDS, dried	1 oz	161	14	2.5	1.5	3	1	1	1	0	+
Planters, dry roasted	1 oz	180	15	2.5	1.5	2	0	1	0	2	+
SWEET POTATOES											
Baked in skin w/salt, medium	1	103	0	0	0	3	8	11500	3	32	0
Green Giant candied, frozen	¾ c	240	7	Na	2.5	3	20	Na	2	20	Na
Green Giant, sweet potato casserole, frozen	1 c	200	10	Na	3	3	17	Na	2	25	Na
SWORDFISH, cooked, dry heat	3 oz	132	4	Na	1	0	0	0	2	1	+
TACO SHELLS, Old El Paso	3 shells	150	7	Na	4	1	0	0	2	0	0
TANGERINE, raw	1 c	103	1	0	0	4	21	302	7	86	0
Minute Maid orange tangerine juice, frozen	1 c	110	0	0	0	0	24	0	35	160	0
POM juice	1 c	140	0	0	0	0	27	0	2	0	0
TEA											
Celestial Seasonings											
All herbal, dessert, holiday, black teas	1 bag	0	0	0	0	0	0	0	0	0	0
Cinnamon spice teahouse chai	3 tbs	110	0	0	0	0	23	Na	15	0	0
Sweet coconut thai chai	3 tbs	110	0	0	0	0	22	Na	10	0	0
Vanilla ginger chai	3 tbs	110	0	0	0	0	23	Na	15	0	0
Lipton											
Chailatta, original	3 tbs	120	2	Na	0	0	19	Na	8	0	0
Chailatta, vanilla	3 tbs	120	2	Na	0	0	19	Na	8	0	0
Hot tea, black or green	1 bag	0	0	0	0	0	0	0	0	0	0

Food	Portion Size	Calories	Total Fat (g)	Good Fats (g)	Bad Fats (g)	Fiber (g)	Sugars (mg)	Beta-carotene (mcg)	Calcium (%DV)	Vit. C (%DV)	B vit. (0,+,++)
Iced green tea w/citrus	8 oz	80	0	0	0	0	21	0	0	0	0
Iced tea mix, sweetened, lemon	1/3 tbs	70	0	0	0	0	18	Na	0	0	0
Iced tea mix, sweetened, raspberry	1½ tbs	80	0	0	0	0	19	Na	0	10	0
Original iced tea, bottles	8 oz	70	0	0	0	0	18	0	0	0	0
TEMPEH											
Lightlife, organic flax	4 oz	220	9	Na	1.5	20	0	Na	0	0	Na
Lightlife, organic garden veggie	4 oz	200	10	Na	1.5	14	0	Na	0	0	Na
Lightlife, organic, three grain	4 oz	230	9	Na	1.5	8	0	Na	0	0	Na
Lightlife organic, wild rice	4 oz	230	7	Na	1	12	0	Na	0	0	Na
TOFU											
Fresh Tofu Inc.											
Baked stuffed	1 pc	160	4.5	Na	0.5	6	0	Na	0	2	Na
Organic baked	2 oz	90	6	Na	6	0	0	Na	4	2	Na
Mori-Nu											
Chinese spice seasoned	3 oz	50	2	Na	0	0	1	0	4	0	0
Japanese miso seasoned	3 oz	60	2.5	Na	0	0	2	0	4	0	0
Silken, extra firm	3 oz	48	1.5	Na	0	0	1	0	2	0	0
Silken, lite extra firm	3 oz	35	0.5	0	0	0	0	0	3	0	0
Silken, soft	3 oz	45	2.5	0.5	0	0	1	0	2	0	0
Nasoya											
Chinese spice firm	¼ pkg	90	5	1	1	1	<1	0	4	0	0
Extra firm	⅕ pkg	80	4.5	1	0.5	1	0	0	6	0	0
Garlic & onion	¼ pkg	90	5	1	1	1	<1	0	4	0	0

Food	Portion Size	Calories	Total Fat (g)	Good Fats (g)	Bad Fats (g)	Fiber (g)	Sugars (mg)	Beta-carotene (mcg)	Calcium (%DV)	Vit. C (%DV)	B vit. (0,+,++)
Lite firm	1/4 pkg	40	1.5	0	0	<1	0	0	15	0	0
Silken	1/5 pkg	45	2	0.5	1	<1	0	0	6	0	0
Soft	1/5 pkg	60	3	0.5	1	<1	0	0	10	0	0
TOMATOES											
Fresh, red, cooked	1 c	43	0	0	0	2	6	703	2	91	0
Fresh, red cherry	1 c	31	0	0	0	2	6	0	0	64	0
Fresh, red, medium	1	26	0	0	0	1	0	0	0	53	0
Fresh, red plum	1	13	0	0	0	1	0	0	0	26	0
Fresh, yellow, chopped	1 c	21	0	0	0	1	0	0	1	20	0
Canned											
Del Monte, diced w/garlic & onion	1/2 c	40	0.5	0	0	<1	6	Na	2	15	0
Del Monte, diced pasta style	1/2 c	45	0	0	0	2	8	Na	2	15	0
Del Monte, stewed, Mexican	1/2 c	35	0	0	0	2	7	130*	2	15	0
Del Monte, wedges	1/2 c	35	0	0	0	2	7	130*	2	15	0
Eden Organic, crushed w/basil	1/4 c	20	0	0	0	1	2	Na	2	15	0
Eden Organic, diced w/green chilis	1/2 c	30	0	0	0	2	3	Na	2	15	0
Eden Organic, whole roma	1/2 c	30	0	0	0	1	2	Na	0	35	0
Muir Glen, diced w/Italian herbs	1/2 c	30	0	0	0	1	3	Na	2	35	0
Muir Glen, whole, fire roasted	1/2 c	25	0	0	0	1	3	Na	2	25	0
Muir Glen, whole, peeled plum	1/2 c	25	0	0	0	1	3	Na	2	30	0
Progresso, crushed	1/4 c	20	0	0	0	0	2	Na	2	10	0
Progresso, diced w/Italian herbs	1/2 c	40	0	0	0	1	6	Na	4	30	0
Progresso, whole peeled w/basil	1/2 c	20	0	0	0	1	3	Na	2	15	0

Food	Portion Size	Calories	Total Fat (g)	Good Fats (g)	Bad Fats (g)	Fiber (g)	Sugars (mg)	Beta-carotene (mcg)	Calcium (%DV)	Vit. C (%DV)	B vit. (0,+,++)
TOMATO JUICE											
Campbell's Healthy Request	8 oz	50	0	0	0	2	9	650*	2	120	+
Campbell's, original	8 oz	50	0	0	0	2	7	650*	2	120	+
TOMATO PASTE/PUREE											
Hunt's, paste	2 tbs	25	0	0	0	2	4	280*	0	10	0
Hunt's, paste, w/basil, garlic, oregano	2 tbs	25	0	0	0	2	4	280*	0	8	0
Hunt's, puree	4 oz	30	0	0	0	2	4	350*	6	30	0
Muir Glen, paste	2 tbs	30	0	0	0	1	3	280*	0	10	0
Muir Glen, puree	1/4 c	25	0	0	0	1	4	350*	0	10	0
Progresso puree	1/4 c	25	0	0	0	1	3	350*	0	10	0
TOPPINGS, DESSERT											
Cool Whip, French vanilla	2 tbs	25	1.5	0	1.5	0	1	0	0	0	0
Cool Whip, lite	2 tbs	20	1	0	1	0	1	0	0	0	0
Cool Whip, regular	2 tbs	25	1.5	0	1.5	2	1	0	0	0	0
Cool Whip, sugar free	2 tbs	20	1	0	1	0	0	0	0	0	0
Smuckers, butterscotch caramel	2 tbs	140	1	0	0.5	0	19	0	6	0	0
Smuckers, Dove dark chocolate	2 tbs	130	4.5	Na	1.5	1	18	0	0	0	0
Smuckers, special recipe hot fudge	2 tbs	130	4.5	Na	1.5	<1	16	0	6	0	0
Smuckers, Spoonable, pecans in syrup	2 tbs	160	9	Na	1	0	15	0	0	0	0
Smuckers, Sundae Syrup, butterscotch	2 tbs	100	0	0	0	0	20	0	2	0	0
Smuckers, Sundae Syrup, caramel	2 tbs	100	0	0	0	0	20	0	2	0	0
TUNA											
Chicken of the Sea											
Chunk, lite in oil	2 oz	110	6	2	1	0	0	0	0	0	+

Food	Portion Size	Calories	Total Fat (g)	Good Fats (g)	Bad Fats (g)	Fiber (g)	Sugars (mg)	Beta-carotene (mcg)	Calcium (%DV)	Vit. C (%DV)	B vit. (0,+,++)
Chunk lite in water	2 oz	60	0.5	0	0	0	0	0	0	0	+
Chunk white in water	2 oz	60	1	0	0	0	0	0	0	0	+
Genova tonno in olive oil	2 oz	130	8	Na	1	0	0	0	0	0	+
Premium, albacore, pouch	2 oz	60	1	0	0	0	0	0	0	0	+
Solid white albacore, in oil	2 oz	90	3	Na	1	0	0	0	0	0	+
Solid white albacore in water	2 oz	70	1	0	0	0	0	0	0	0	+
Starkist											
Chunk light pouch	3 oz	90	1	0	0	0	0	0	0	0	+
Chunk light water	2 oz	60	0.5	0	0	0	0	0	0	0	+
Gourmet choice fillet, water	2 oz	60	1	0	0	0	0	0	0	0	+
Solid white albacore, water	2 oz	70	1	0	0	0	0	0	0	0	+
TURKEY											
Dark meat, roasted, diced	1 c	261	10	2	3	0	0	0	4	0	+
Giblets, cooked, chopped	1 c	288	17	7	6	0	0	0	2	33	++
Light meat, roasted, diced	1 c	219	5	1	1	0	0	0	2	0	+
Louis Rich, pure ground	4 oz	180	11	Na	3.5	0	0	0	2	0	+
Roast, boneless, frozen, roasted, diced	1 c	209	8	1.5	3	0	0	0	0	0	+
TURNIPS, cooked, no salt, cubes	1 c	34	0	0	0	3	5	0	5	30	0
TURNIP GREENS, chopped, cooked	1 c	28	0	0	0	5	1	6588	19	65	+
VEAL											
Breast, boneless, lean	3 oz	185	8	4	3	0	0	0	0	0	+
Leg, lean	3 oz	128	3	1	1	0	0	0	0	0	+
Loin, lean	3 oz	149	6	2	2	0	0	0	1	0	+

Food	Portion Size	Calories	Total Fat (g)	Good Fats (g)	Bad Fats (g)	Fiber (g)	Sugars (mg)	Beta-carotene (mcg)	Calcium (%DV)	Vit. C (%DV)	B vit. (0,+,++)
Rib, lean	3 oz	185	7	2	2	0	0	0	2	0	+
Sirloin, lean	3 oz	143	5	2	2	0	0	0	1	0	+
VEGETABLE JUICE											
Knudsen, Very Veggie low sodium	8 oz	50	0	0	0	2	2	2000*	2	10	0
Knudsen, Very Veggie, original	8 oz	50	0	0	0	2	7	2000*	2	20	0
Knudsen, Very Veggie, spicy	8 oz	50	0	0	0	2	7	2000*	2	20	0
V-8 calcium enriched	8 oz	80	0	0	0	3	12	2000*	45	180	0
V-8, low sodium	8 oz	50	0	0	0	2	8	2000*	2	120	0
V-8 picante	8 oz	50	0	0	0	2	8	2000*	4	120	0
V-8, 100%	8 oz	50	0	0	0	2	8	2000*	4	120	0
VEGETABLES, mixed											
Canned											
Del Monte, home style medley	½ c	70	2.5	Na	0	2	3	Na	4	8	Na
Del Monte mixed	½ c	40	0	0	0	2	3	Na	2	4	Na
Del Monte mixed w/potatoes	½ c	45	0	0	0	2	3	Na	4	10	Na
S&W, mixed	½ c	45	0	0	0	2	3	Na	4	10	Na
Birds Eye											
Asian in sesame ginger	1 c	60	1	0	0	2	0	Na	2	15	Na
Baby corn & vegetable blend	⅔ c	50	1	0	0	3	0	Na	2	10	Na
Baby pea & vegetable blend	¾ c	40	0	0	0	2	0	Na	2	8	Na
Baby potato & vegetable blend	¾ c	40	0	0	0	1	0	Na	2	15	Na
California blend & cheddar cheese	½ c	80	4	Na	2	1	0	Na	6	35	Na
Classic mixed	⅔ c	60	0	0	0	2	0	Na	2	6	Na

Food	Portion Size	Calories	Total Fat (g)	Good Fats (g)	Bad Fats (g)	Fiber (g)	Sugars (mg)	Beta-carotene (mcg)	Calcium (%DV)	Vit. C (%DV)	B vit. (0,+,++)
Szechuan in sesame sauce	1 c	60	2	Na	0	2	0	Na	2	25	Na
Tuscan vegetables in herbed tomato	1 c	50	2	Na	0	2	0	Na	2	10	Na
Cascadian Farm											
California style blend	⅔ c	25	0	0	0	2	2	Na	2	25	Na
Chinese stir fry	1 c	25	0	0	0	2	2	Na	2	20	Na
Garden's blend	¾ c	50	0	0	0	2	4	Na	0	6	Na
Thai stir fry	¾ c	25	0	0	0	2	2	Na	2	20	Na
Green Giant											
Baby vegetable medley	¾ c	60	2	Na	1	2	4	Na	2	20	Na
Boxed alfredo	¾ c	40	1	0	0	8	4	Na	6	30	Na
Garden medley, prep.	½ c	70	0.5	0	0	2	3	Na	2	25	Na
Plain mixed, prep.	½ c	50	0	0	0	2	3	Na	0	6	Na
Simply steam garden medley, prep.	½ c	50	0.5	0	0	1	3	Na	2	20	Na
Szechuan vegetables	¾ c	50	0.5	0	0	2	5	Na	2	35	Na
Teriyaki vegetables	1¼ c	70	4.5	Na	2	2	4	Na	2	35	Na
VINEGAR											
Eden Foods, apple cider or red wine organic	1 tbs	0	0	0	0	0	1	0	0	0	0
Eden Foods, brown rice, organic	1 tbs	2	0	0	0	0	0	0	0	0	0
Eden Foods, ume plum, imported	1 tbs	0	0	0	0	0	0	0	0	0	0
WAFFLES–see "Frozen Breakfast," "Pancakes & Waffles"											

Food	Portion Size	Calories	Total Fat (g)	Good Fats (g)	Bad Fats (g)	Fiber (g)	Sugars (mg)	Beta-carotene (mcg)	Calcium (%DV)	Vit. C (%DV)	B vit. (0,+,++)
WALNUTS											
Black, dried	1 oz	175	17	4	1	2	0	7	1	0	0
English	1 oz	183	18	2.5	2	2	1	3	2	0	0
Planters	1 oz	210	20	Na	2	2	1	7*	4	2	0
WATER CHESTNUTS, raw	½ c	60	0	0	0	2	3	0	4	4	0
WATERMELON, balls	1 c	46	0	0	0	1	10	466	1	20	0
WHITEFISH, cooked	3 oz	146	6	2	1	0	0	0	2	0	+
Smoked	3 oz	92	1	0	0	0	0	0	1	0	+
WINE											
Red table (average values)	5 oz	125	0	0	0	0	0	0	0	0	0
Rose table (average values)	3 oz	73	0	0	0	0	0	0	0	0	0
White table (average values)	5 oz	122	0	0	0	0	0	0	0	0	0
YAM, boiled or baked, cubes	1 c	158	0	0	0	5	1	99	1	27	0
Canned, candied (S&W)	½ c	170	0	0	0	4	21	Na	2	8	Na
YOGURT											
Columbo											
Classic banana strawberry	8 oz	230	2	Na	1.5	0	42	Na	20	0	+
Classic blueberry, cherry, peach, raspberry, strawberry	8 oz	220	2	Na	1.5	0	36	Na	20	0	++
Classic vanilla	8 oz	190	2.5	Na	1.5	0	27	Na	25	0	++
Light: blueberry, cherry vanilla, key lime, mixed berry, peach, raspberry, strawberry	8 oz	120	0	0	0	0	15	Na	35	0	+
Low fat, plain	8 oz	100	0	0	0	0	10	Na	30	0	++
Low fat, strawberry or vanilla	8 oz	220	2.5	Na	1.5	0	34	Na	25	0	++

Food	Portion Size	Calories	Total Fat (g)	Good Fats (g)	Bad Fats (g)	Fiber (g)	Sugars (mg)	Beta-carotene (mcg)	Calcium (%DV)	Vit. C (%DV)	B vit. (0,+,++)
Dannon											
Activia, prune	4 oz	110	2	Na	1	0	17	Na	15	0	+
Activia, strawberry	4 oz	110	2	Na	1	0	17	Na	15	0	+
Activia, vanilla	4 oz	110	2	Na	1.5	0	17	Na	15	0	+
DanActive, blueberry, cranberry/raspberry, strawberry, or vanilla	3.3 oz	90	1.5	0	1	0	17	Na	10	0	0
DanActive, plain	3.3 oz	90	1.5	0	1.5	0	15	Na	10	0	0
Fruit on Bottom, apple cinnamon	6 oz	150	1.5	0	1	<1	25	Na	20	2	+
Fruit on Bottom, cherry	6 oz	140	1.5	0	1	0	24	Na	20	4	+
Fruit on Bottom, mixed berry	6 oz	150	1.5	0	1.5	<1	27	Na	20	4	+
Fruit on Bottom, pineapple	6 oz	150	1.5	0	1.5	0	27	Na	20	4	+
Frusion, cherry berry blend	10 oz	260	3.5	Na	2	<1	47	Na	25	4	+
Frusion, pina colada	10 oz	260	3.5	Na	2	0	48	Na	25	4	+
Frusion, strawberry blend	10 oz	260	3.5	Na	2	0	48	Na	25	4	+
La Crème, all flavors	4 oz	140	5	Na	3	0	18	Na	15	0	+
Stonyfield											
Cultured O'Soy, blueberry	6 oz	170	2	Na	0	4	27	Na	15	0	0
Cultured O'Soy, chocolate	6 oz	160	3	Na	0	4	22	Na	10	0	0
Cultured O'Soy, vanilla	6 oz	150	2	Na	0	4	21	Na	15	0	0
Fat-free, apricot mango	6 oz	130	0	0	0	2	23	Na	30	0	0
Fat-free, chocolate underground	6 oz	170	0	0	0	3	34	Na	30	0	0
Fat-free French vanilla	6 oz	180	0	0	0	2	25	Na	35	0	0
Fat-free, lotsa lemon	6 oz	140	0	0	0	2	25	Na	35	0	0

Food	Portion Size	Calories	Total Fat (g)	Good Fats (g)	Bad Fats (g)	Fiber (g)	Sugars (mg)	Beta-carotene (mcg)	Calcium (%DV)	Vit. C (%DV)	B vit. (0,+,++)
Fat-free, peach	6 oz	120	0	0	0	2	23	Na	30	0	0
Fat-free, plain	8 oz	100	0	0	0	2	12	Na	35	0	0
Smoothies, reg, banana berry	10 oz	250	3	Na	2	4	41	Na	40	0	+
Smoothies, reg, strawberry or vanilla	10 oz	250	3	Na	2	4	41	Na	40	0	+
Smoothies, light, banana berry	10 oz	130	0	0	0	3	20	Na	25	0	0
Smoothies, light, peach	10 oz	130	0	0	0	3	19	Na	25	2	0
Smoothies, light, strawberry	10 oz	130	0	0	0	3	19	Na	25	2	0
Yoplait											
Go-Gurt, smoothies, all flavors, bottle	1	120	0.5	Na	0	0	20	Na	20	0	Na
Grande, all flavors	8 oz	220	2.5	Na	1.5	0	34	Na	25	0	+
Grande, plain, fat free	8 oz	130	0	0	0	0	17	Na	40	0	+
Grande, light, all flavors	8 oz	140	0	0	0	0	22	Na	25	0	‡
Nouriche, all flavors	1 cont	260	0	0	0	5	22	Na	30	25	+
Original, most flavors	6 oz	170	1.5	Na	1	0	27	Na	20	0	+
Original, coconut cream	6 oz	190	3	0	2	0	27	Na	20	0	+
Original, pina colada	6 oz	170	2	0	1.5	0	28	Na	20	0	+
Original, plain	6 oz	100	0	0	0	0	13	Na	20	0	+
Smoothie, light, all flavors	8 oz	90	0	0	0	3	0	Na	20	0	+
Smoothie, all flavors	8 oz	190	2.5	Na	1.5	3	31	Na	20	0	+
Thick & creamy, all flavors, low fat	6 oz	190	3.5	Na	2	0	28	Na	30	0	Na
Whips! All chocolate flavors	4 oz	160	4	Na	2.5	0	23	Na	10	0	Na
Whips! All other flavors	4 oz	140	2.5	0	2	0	21	Na	15	0	Na

Food	Portion Size	Calories	Total Fat (g)	Good Fats (g)	Bad Fats (g)	Fiber (g)	Sugars (mg)	Beta-carotene (mcg)	Calcium (%DV)	Vit. C (%DV)	B vit. (0,+,++)
YOGURT, frozen											
Ben & Jerry's											
Cherry Garcia, low fat	½ c	170	3	Na	2	<1	22	Na	20	0	0
Chocolate fudge brownie, low fat	½ c	190	2.5	Na	1.5	1	23	Na	15	0	0
Half baked, low fat	½ c	190	3	Na	1.5	<1	23	Na	15	0	0
Phish food	½ c	220	4.5	Na	3.5	1	22	Na	15	0	0
Häagen-Dazs											
Coffee	½ c	200	4.5	Na	2.5	0	20	Na	20	0	0
Vanilla, low fat	½ c	200	4.5	Na	2.5	0	21	Na	25	0	0
Vanilla raspberry swirl	½ c	170	2.5	Na	1.5	0	24	Na	10	2	0
Wildberry	½ c	180	2	Na	1	0	27	Na	15	6	0
Stonyfield											
After dark chocolate, organic, nonfat	½ c	100	0	0	0	0	18	Na	15	0	0
Cookies 'n cream, low fat	½ c	130	1	Na	0	0	19	Na	15	0	0
Gotta have vanilla, organic, nonfat	½ c	100	0	0	0	0	19	Na	15	0	0
Javalanche, organic, nonfat	½ c	100	0	0	0	0	18	Na	15	0	0
Vanilla fudge swirl	½ c	120	0	0	0	0	22	Na	15	0	0
ZUCCHINI, cooked, no salt, slices	1 c	29	0	0	0	2	4	1200	1	6	0
Raw, w/skin	1 c	20	0	0	0	1	2	135	1	32	0
Canned, w/tomato (Del Monte)	½ c	30	0	0	0	1	1	0	0	4	0

REFERENCES

CHAPTER 1

Institutes of Medicine website: http://www.iom
.edu/Object.File/Master/21/372/0.pdf.

National Institutes of Arthritis and Musculoskeletal and Skin Diseases website: http://www.niams.
nih.gov/bone/hi/overview.htm.

Quadri, P, et al. Homocysteine and B vitamins in
mild cognitive impairment and dementia. *Clin
Chem Lab Med* 43(10):1,096–1,100, 2005.

Snowdon, DA, et al. Linguistic ability in early life
and cognitive function and Alzheimer's disease
in late life. Findings from the Nun Study. *JAMA*
275(7):528–532, 1996.

Vlassara, H, et al. Inflammatory mediators are in-
duced by dietary glycotoxins, a major risk factor
for diabetic angiopathy. *Proc Natl Acad Sci USA*
99(24):15,596–15,601, 2002.

Wilson, RS, et al. Participation in cognitively stim-
ulating activities and risk of incident Alzheimer's disease. *JAMA* 287:742–748, 2002.

CHAPTER 2

Asami, DK, et al. Comparison of the total phenolic
and ascorbic content of freeze-dried and air-
dried marionberry, strawberry, and corn grown
using conventional, organic, and sustainable
agricultural practices. *J Agric Food Chem* 51(5):
1237–1241, 2003.

Caris-Veyvat, C, et al. Influence of organic versus
conventional agricultural practice on the antioxidant microconstituent content of tomatoes
and derived purees; consequences on antioxidant
plasma status in humans. *J Agric Food Chem*
52(21):6,503–6,509, 2004.

Fife, Bruce ND. *The Detox Book* (Colorado Springs:
HealthWise, 1997).

Food Additives and Contaminants, May 8, 2002.

Worthington, V. Nutritional quality of organic versus conventional fruits, vegetables, and grains.
J Altern Comple Med 7(2):161–173, 2001.

CHAPTER 3

Albert, CM, et al. Nut consumption and decreased
risk of sudden cardiac death in the Physicians'
Health Study. *Arch Intern Med* 162(12):1,382–
1,387, 2002.

Cabrera, C, et al. Beneficial effects of green tea—a review. *J Am Coll Nutr* 25(2):79–99, 2006.

Dandona, P, et al. Inflammation: the link between insulin resistance, obesity, and diabetes. *Trends Immunol* 25(1):4–7, 2004.

Dills, WL. Protein fructosylation: fructose and the Maillard reaction. *Am J Clin Nutr* 58 (Suppl):779–875, 1993.

Fleming, RM. The effect of high-protein diets on coronary blood flow. *Angiology* 51(10):817–826, 2000.

Haas, Elson M, MD. Nutritional program for anti-aging. At http://www.healthy.net/scr/article.asp?ID=1272#2.

Kelly, JH Jr., Sabate, J. Nuts and coronary heart disease: an epidemiological perspective. *Br J Nutr* 96 (Suppl 2):S61–S67, 2006.

Maher, JH. Phytonutrients, lifelong wellness and the theories of aging. *JAAIM*. At http://www.aaimedicine.com/jaaim/oct05/phytonutrients2.php.

Mayo Clinic. Water: How much should you drink every day? At http://www.mayoclinic.com/health/water/NU00283.

Nakagawa, T, et al. Protective activity of green tea against free radical- and glucose-mediated protein damage. *J Agricul Food Chem* 50(8):2418–2422, 2002.

Owen, RW, et al. Olive-oil consumption and health: the possible role of antioxidants. *Lancet Oncol* 107–112, 2000.

Sabate, J. Nut consumption, vegetarian diets, ischemic heart disease risk, and all-cause mortality: evidence from epidemiologic studies. *Am J Clin Nutr* 70(Suppl 3):500S–503S, 1999.

Shannon, J, et al. Relationship of food groups and water intake to colon cancer risk. *Cancer Epidemiology Biomarkers and Prevention* 5(7):495–502, 1996.

Simopoulos, A. Omega-3 fatty acids in inflammation and autoimmune diseases. *J Am Coll Nutr* (6):495–505, 2002.